Coping with Endometriosis

Coping with Endometriosis

Bringing Compassion to Pain, Shame and Uncertainty

Dr Kirsty Harris

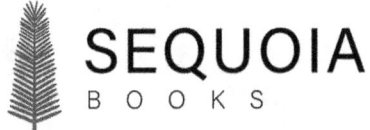

Every possible effort has been made to ensure that the information contained in this book is accurate at the time of going to press. The publishers and author(s) cannot accept responsibility for any errors and omissions, however caused. No responsibility for loss or damage occasioned to any person acting, or refraining from action, as a result of the material contained in this publication can be accepted by the editor, the publisher or the author.

First published in 2024 by Sequoia Books

Apart from fair dealing for the purposes of research or private study, or criticism or review, as permitted under the Copyright, Designs and Patents act 1988, this publication may only be reproduced, stored or transmitted, in any form or by any means, with the prior permission in writing of the publisher, or in the case of reprographic reproduction in accordance with the terms and licenses issued by the CLA. Enquiries concerning reproduction outside these terms should be sent to the publisher using the details on the website www.sequoia-books.com

©Kirsty Harris 2024

The right of Dr Kirsty Harris to be identified as author of this work has been asserted in accordance with the Copyright, Designs and Patents act 1988.

ISBN
Print: 9781914110344
EPUB: 9781914110351

A CIP record for this book is available from the British Library

Library of Congress Cataloguing-In-Publication Data

Name: Kirsty Harris
Title: Coping With Endometriosis/Harris
Description: 1st Edition, Sequoia Books UK 2024
Print: 9781914110344
EPUB: 9781914110351

Library of Congress Control Number: 2024903214

Print and Electronic production managed by Deanta Global

To women and menstruating people everywhere – know your experience is real, that it matters and that you are not alone. Together we can make a difference and change will happen.

To my daughter, you are my reason to fight for change. I love you.

Contents

Foreword	xi
The Unique Perspective	xii
Acknowledgements	xiv

1	**An Introduction to Me and My Journey**	1
	Introduction	1
	My Family	2
	My Education and Career	4
	My 'Problem Periods'	6
2	**Understanding Menstrual Health and Endometriosis**	19
	What Is Menstrual Health?	20
	The Menstrual Cycle: Medical Phases and Changing Seasons	24
	Menstrual Tracking	27
	Endometriosis and Other Gynaecological Conditions	30
	What Is Endometriosis?	31
	Endometriosis: Prevalence, Signs, Symptoms, and Classification	31
	Endometriosis Classification	34
	Other Gynaecological Conditions	36
	Endometriosis Treatments	38
	Summary	40
3	**A Psychological Understanding of Endometriosis Using Compassion-Focussed Therapy (CFT)**	41
	Psychological Thinking and Formulation	41

Compassion-Focussed Therapy (CFT)	46
The 'Tricky Brain'	49
Understanding Tricky Loops	50
The Three-Systems Model	52
Threat and Self-Protection System	53
The Drive System	54
Soothing and Contentment System	54
The Compassionate Mind	55
Mapping Your Own Systems	56
Summary	60
4 What Is Compassion and Why Is It Difficult?	**61**
What Is Compassion?	61
Qualities of Compassion	62
The Flows of Compassion	65
Barriers to Compassion	67
Understanding the Origins of Our Fears and Their Unintended Consequences	71
Introduction to Skills	73
Summary	75
5 Understanding Threat	**77**
The Body's Response to Threat	77
Triggering the Threat Response	80
Threat Responses – Strategies to Keep Us Safe in Response to Threat	82
Trauma and the Body	86
Connecting with Threat in Our Bodies	88
Soothing Rhythm Breathing	90
Summary	92
6 Understanding Shame and Its Relevance in Endometriosis	**94**
What Is Shame?	94
Why Is Shame a Threat to Us?	95

	Where Does Shame Come From and Why Do We Experience Shame?	96
	Body Shame and Endometriosis	101
	Not Naming and Shaming – Naming and Taming!	104
	Naming Shame in Ourselves	107
	Bringing Compassion to Shame	109
	Summary	109
7	Endometriosis and Your Relationship with Yourself	111
	Understanding Your Own Self-Criticism and Self-Critic	112
	Imagining the Self-Critic	114
	Developing a Compassionate Self	117
	Connecting with the Self-to-Self Flow of Compassion	122
	Compassionate Self-Correction	124
	Summary	126
8	Endometriosis and Relationships	127
	How Endometriosis Impacts Relationships	127
	Endometriosis at Work	130
	Endometriosis and Friendships	133
	Endometriosis and Romantic Relationships	134
	Sex and Intimacy	137
	Talking about Endometriosis with Others: The Search for Support	139
	Receiving Compassion from Others	141
	Developing a Compassionate Other	144
	Being Assertive	146
	Summary	149
9	Relationship with Endometriosis	151
	Introduction	151
	Endometriosis and Fertility	151
	Fertility and Managing Difficult Emotions	155
	Endometriosis, Persistent Pain, and Disability	158
	Compassionate Behaviour	163

Using the Compassionate Self to Work with Difficulties	165
Making Changes	166
Using Compassion to Make Decisions about Treatment	169
Summary	174
10 A Commitment to Compassion	**175**
Connecting with Compassion – An Ongoing Commitment	176
My Own Commitment to Connecting with Compassion	178
Your Commitment to Connecting with Compassion	181
How to Get More Support	183
Resources	183
Mental Health Concerns	183
If you are at risk to yourself	186
Resources for Endometriosis and Other Gynaecological Conditions	187
CFT Resources	187
Relationship Support and Resources	187
Employment Support and Resources	187
Fertility Support and Resources	188
Baby Loss Charities	188
References	189
About the Author	194

Foreword

Dr Sarah Swan
Coping with ... Series Editor
Consultant Clinical Psychologist

When I was diagnosed with breast cancer in 2019, I knew I was going to have to use my skills as a clinical psychologist to help me cope with the distress that this inevitably caused. Early on in my journey, I had the urge to write, as a way of processing my experiences. I immediately thought it had the potential for a book, but never thought this would come to fruition. But with the support of the Association of Clinical Psychologists, Sequoia Publishing, friends, family, and colleagues, I committed to writing the book.

I began to realise what a unique position I held; facing a difficult life event that many others face, but with the knowledge and experience of a long career in helping people with their emotional experiences. Suddenly, it dawned on me that there could be any number of difficult or challenging experiences that other clinical psychologists may have faced. And, like me, they would in all likelihood have valuable skills to share with others facing the same situation. And so, the idea for the series was born.

It is an honour to launch the series with my book, *Coping with Breast Cancer*. And it has been my pleasure to support other clinical psychologists with their writing in order to produce a series of books that will help to bring valuable psychological ideas to a wide audience. With the knowledge and skills of the writers, I am confident that this series will benefit many people facing difficult and challenging situations and give them helpful skills to cope.

The Unique Perspective

Dr Penelope Cream
Clinical & Health Psychologist
Director of Operations, ACP-UK

The Association of Clinical Psychologists (ACP-UK) is delighted to be publishing these important *Coping with …* books. In these pages clinical psychologists have taken the courageous step of sharing how they applied their skills to their own lives, in order to help others facing similar difficulties and challenges.

The profession of clinical psychology spans many types of psychological approach across all areas of the lifespan and of individual experiences, from physical health, psychological distress, and mental illness, as well as cognitive difficulties, family challenges, and workplace problems. Clinical psychologists have rigorous training not only in psychological therapies but also in research methods and using evidence-based practice. They draw on these aspects to inform everything they do, including looking after themselves. These books evidence the flexibility and creativity with which we can use and apply our skills, both to help ourselves and others.

It is not often that clinicians share their first-hand experiences of challenging situations and how they have applied what they have learnt in their training and the many years of experience that follow. I feel very proud of my clinical psychology colleagues who have written this series of books, not only for everything that they have experienced

The Unique Perspective

with courage and insight, but for the generosity and openness with which they want to help other people. It is not easy to combine subjective personal experience with an external clinical perspective, yet in these books they share the breadth of knowledge and training that the profession brings us.

Acknowledgements

There are many people who have supported me and helped me to cope with the impact endometriosis has had on my life. It would be impossible to acknowledge everyone who has had an impact on my journey and made it better. To anyone who took the time to ask what they could do to help me, to everyone who listened and those who changed things with me or for me, I am thankful to you all.

Although I cannot thank everyone here, there are some people who I want to mention. Tom, your support means this book is a reality and when I doubt myself it is your voice that reminds me, I can do this. Helen, for listening endlessly and never making me feel like it was any trouble to hear me. Dad and Chris, for your support with anything I needed. Mum, for being there throughout my journey and never giving up on trying to help me find a way though this. Nan, for showing me anything is possible and never letting me give up. To all my family and friends who have showed endless compassion and understanding, I love you all.

Sarah Swan and ACP-UK who have supported this book and the series, giving me the opportunity to make something that started as a nice idea into a reality. Thank you to those who read and or provided support on my early draft: Tom, Mum, Laura Johnson @thetroublewithendo, Natalie @honestlyendo, Christie Lee @endometriosis.dietician, Anna @battlewithendo_ox and Anna and Gabi @themenstrualhealthproject.

I want to also thank Paul Gilbert, Hannah Gilbert and The Compassionate Mind Foundation for their dedication to CFT, which has been so helpful to me. Also to Deborah Lee, Chris Irons, and Michelle Cree who have inspired me with their teaching and books.

Acknowledgements

And finally, to David. You have lived this with me, and I cannot imagine doing it without you. You have also given me the time to share my story, and some of yours, in this book and I hope that makes a difference for many other couples like us.

1 An Introduction to Me and My Journey

Introduction

I want to start this book by introducing myself, my journey, and my motivation for sharing my experience with you. If you have bought this book, or you're considering buying it and reading this first paragraph in a bookstore, then chances are you are someone, or you care about someone, with endometriosis or symptoms of it. Endometriosis is estimated to affect 190 million people worldwide (WHO, 2023), and it can take eight years to receive a diagnosis (Endometriosis UK). In 2021 aged 33, I had a hysterectomy and excision (removal) of severe endometriosis. It was widespread throughout my pelvis, had damaged my ovaries, and had begun to infiltrate my bowel. The decision to have a hysterectomy, knowing this was not a cure for endometriosis, was one of the most difficult ones I have made in my life. I had suffered from gynaecological problems since I was 12 years old, and they had gradually come to dominate my life and disable me in a variety of ways. It took 20 years for me to receive a confirmed diagnosis of endometriosis and adenomyosis.

Alongside the physical impact that endometriosis had on me, it also had many psychological and emotional consequences that I did not fully understand at the time. It impacted my relationship with myself and my relationships with others. It stole parts of my life and left me grieving for what I had lost. It influenced every part of my world, and no one talked to me about that or how to cope with it. Over the years, I was able to make sense of this using compassion-focused therapy which I learnt in my training as a clinical psychologist. This model by Paul Gilbert and the work of his colleagues at the Compassionate Mind Foundation enabled me to make sense of my experience and learn how to connect differently with my suffering. I want to share how I have applied this model and concepts from Paul Gilbert's work to my own experience in the hope that it will be helpful to you.

I do not claim to speak for everyone with endometriosis. Nor am I suggesting that the ways I coped and the decisions I made are the right ones. However, I hope that sharing my personal experience and how this was influenced by my professional knowledge and training will be helpful to others navigating the challenges of the condition.

My Family

I was born in the midlands in the UK right at the end of 1987 – New Year's Eve to be precise and no, it's not a good day to have a birthday. When I was born, the midwife announced, 'you have a beautiful little girl' and for me, that gender descriptor has been correct. I would be accurately described as a cis-gender, heterosexual woman. I believe this is relevant to discussing the endometriosis journey described in this book, as the experiences of menstruation and its difficulties are often discussed within the context of being a woman and often a heterosexual one. I want you to know that this book is for all people who menstruate. However, you identify and whatever has brought you to this book, know that you are seen and your experience matters. I hope this book is helpful to all of you.

My parents are liberal and open-minded people, and I have always known they only wanted me to be happy and share in my experiences – good and bad. They separated when I was around 18 months old and co-parented throughout my life. Both of my parents worked hard to be open with me about life, including the parts that are difficult. My parents will always listen, and always want to help. Their willingness to listen, to be there in the presence of their own vulnerability and discomfort is something I think they are aspirational in. I am thankful for both of my parents' support throughout my life, but we all recognise now that we lacked knowledge on endometriosis and its impact, and this has been a challenge for us to navigate as a family.

An Introduction to Me and My Journey

I met my husband when I was 21 years old. About three months after meeting him, he was hospitalised due to a short illness and a few months after I had one of the most significant hospital admissions of my life. I remember being in the hospital and feeling like these challenges so early in our relationship felt like something that would make or break us. At the time, neither of us realised how many of those moments we would face as a couple. Looking back now, I don't think endometriosis has 'made' our relationship. Although it may have strengthened our connection with each other in some ways, I also think it has taken things from us and placed us under strain that could have broken us apart. Despite this, when I faced the many challenges I will share in this book, my husband was there by my side. I, like many others, have felt guilty for the impact endometriosis has had on my husband, my daughter, and my wider family. However, we are fortunate as a couple that when we face struggles, we have faced them together, and we have come through them together. My husband is probably the only person in the world who has some understanding of the impact of my illness on me when it was at its worst. Despite this, he says that he could never fully understand what I was going through, and this was apparent at times. Although there were many parts of my experience that made me feel alone, and many decisions that could not be made for me, knowing I had people in my corner regardless was a foundation I could use to help me cope. For some of you, this won't be a partner or a family member, and if this is the case, I hope there are others in your life who can support you and that this book can enable you to connect with people who can offer you compassion.

In 2015, I gave birth to our daughter. She was five years old when I had my excision surgery and hysterectomy. I hope that this means she will not see the worst of my suffering and wanting to be present for her was a significant factor in my decision to have the surgery. I worry about what she might face when she begins menstruating, and she is part of the motivation for this book. I do not want her to experience the journey so many women, including her mother, have experienced before her. I cannot control whether she has endometriosis, but I hope

I can influence changes that mean she never suffers as I did. I hope she never feels alone.

My Education and Career

I loved school. I enjoyed learning and being part of a community. I was 14 years old when I decided I wanted to be a clinical psychologist. On reflection, my interest in psychology came in part from my family and in part from my teachers. My family are all compassionate and accepting people. They are also very resilient, a particular interest of many psychologists all over the world. However, it was my teachers who formally introduced me to the study of people, something which has been my passion ever since.

Becoming a clinical psychologist in the UK requires you to complete an undergraduate course that is accredited by the British Psychological Society and then an accredited doctoral degree in clinical psychology. Obtaining a place on the doctoral course is highly competitive. Historically, there were ratios of five applicants to one place (Roth, 1998). Clinical psychology training is funded by the NHS, meaning you are paid as a trainee clinical psychologist whilst you complete your doctoral degree. You also work in the NHS during this time. There are no fees for the training programme which is different to many other areas of psychology which are self-funded or provide a small bursary rather than a wage (e.g. counselling or forensic psychology). I am mindful that part of the reason I chose clinical psychology was a socio-economic one. I had already accumulated debt as an undergraduate, and I was not able to fund a post-graduate degree. Clinical psychology allowed me the only realistic pathway into the career that I love.

I first studied psychology at A-Level, and I went on to study psychology at Leicester University. I graduated with first-class honours and started my first job as an assistant psychologist. Two years later I was offered a place to complete my Doctorate in Clinical Psychology at the University of Oxford. After training, I worked in acute inpatient and forensic units which I really enjoyed. In 2018, the opportunity to work in a perinatal mental health team presented itself, and I began working in a specialist community perinatal mental health service leading the psychological interventions pathway within the county. Perinatal mental health services provide mental health care during pregnancy up until two years after birth (Royal College of Psychiatrists, 2021). In 2021, my role expanded to include leading a maternal mental health service, which offers psychological intervention to women and birthing people who have experience perinatal trauma and loss.

I believe some of my interest in perinatal work has been born out of my personal experience. Many of the people I treat now have experienced endometriosis, complex fertility journeys, perinatal loss, and other gynaecological health conditions. Part of the reason I have been able to navigate my personal journey is because of my professional background and training. I have often asked myself 'what would you say if you were your own therapist?' and separated out the clinical psychologist in me from just me. Without that ability and education, I think I would have had a very different journey, and I believe my mental health would have suffered considerably.

Although my personal experience has drawn me to the work I do and helps me to understand the experience of the people I treat, it is often not something I share in my role as a clinical psychologist. Personal disclosure must be carefully considered in a therapeutic relationship, and I tend to feel that therapy is not the place to share my own journey or experience. However, I do believe that it could be helpful to others, and I can think of many times I have wanted to share it with people I have treated.

When the opportunity came along to write this book, it seemed like an ideal time to share how the clinical psychologist within me has helped me to survive the challenges I have faced in relation to my menstrual and gynaecological health. I intentionally use the word survival as I cannot claim to have coped or overcome the challenges endometriosis has thrown at me. I began my journey with endometriosis long before I became a clinical psychologist. I had learnt to cope in ways that might not have been helpful for me. I also didn't understand what was happening to me for decades. Through my professional training, I have learnt about multiple different therapies, including skills which have been helpful to me, in particular compassion-focussed therapy. This book is based on the work of Paul Gilbert and the Compassionate Mind Foundation which I have learnt about and used in my professional role. I am grateful to the Compassionate Mind Foundation, Professor Gilbert, and all of the other psychologists and psychological therapists who have made this work accessible to others.

As my professional knowledge developed, and my inner clinical psychologist had suggestions on what might be helpful, I haven't always listened, and many times I have ignored them. It is important to know that as someone who suffers with this condition, sometimes the best you can do is survive. I hope to be able to share with you an honest account of my experience including the highs and the lows. I want to share with you the theories, skills, and ideas developed by Paul Gilbert and others that have been of use to me as I have navigated 20+ years of gynaecological uncertainty and debilitating pain until my diagnosis and hysterectomy in 2021. I hope that they are helpful to you and remind you that you are not alone.

My 'Problem Periods'

For most of my life, my experiences and symptoms were explained as 'problem periods', and there were times I thought the problem might be me. I did not receive a confirmed diagnosis of endometriosis until I had my hysterectomy, 21 years after my periods started. By this time, I had internalised the belief that I was at best part of the problem, at worst I was the problem. I believed that I was incapable of coping with a period and that everyone else was coping better than I was. This was reinforced by my experience of some healthcare professionals, other people in my life, and by wider education and societal beliefs at that time.

When I learnt about periods at school (now called menstrual health education), I didn't learn that some periods are not 'normal' (see chapter 2). I did know what a period was and that I would have them. However, I was given the impression they were a minor inconvenience that would not adversely impact your life in any way. My periods started when I was 12 years old, and they quickly became a problem. Within a year, I had my first admission to hospital connected with 'problem periods'. I also experienced several other health problems that were seen as separate to the period problems, including recurrent urinary tract infections (UTIs), back pain, and leg pain. However, I have since learnt that these are symptoms of endometriosis, and I think this was the link between all my difficulties over the years, but no one joined the dots.

Through this book, I will share the detail of different parts of my experience. However, I also wanted to provide a summary of my experience with this condition from the outset. My intention is to give you an overview of my problem periods from their onset (aged 12) to their end (aged 33) to underpin the rest of the book. The end of my periods does not mark the end of my symptoms or my experience with endometriosis. However, my hysterectomy and the end of my monthly bleed have marked an end point of sorts in that part of my journey.

I have accessed both NHS and private healthcare to seek help with my symptoms. I had positive and negative experiences of healthcare professionals at different times in my journey. Unfortunately, I had more difficult experiences with healthcare professionals than positive ones, but I think this reflected a lack of awareness and understanding of endometriosis at those times. I was fortunate to be able to access private consultants at times during my journey, and I chose to have my hysterectomy surgery privately, partly due to the increased waiting times caused in part by the COVID-19 pandemic. I recognise that being able to access private healthcare is a privilege that is not available to everyone. However, I would have made the same choices and accessed the same surgery via the NHS, so I hope my experience is still valuable even if it is different to your own.

For those of you going through this experience, you will know that summarising the impact of endometriosis is difficult. You repeat your story many times, and parts of it get lost along the way as it becomes so much a part of your daily life you forget it is not 'normal'. I was faced with this same dilemma when I met the consultant who went on to perform my hysterectomy. Although we all hope that our notes have been read, they may not represent our journey the way we would do ourselves. I sat down one evening with my file of medical notes and produced a timeline which I emailed to the consultant in advance of our first appointment.

The table presented below is an anonymised and updated version of that timeline which was completed prior to my hysterectomy and excision surgery. I include this not only to give you an overview of my personal experience, but as an example so that you can use it as a guide or template should you wish to create a similar summary of your own experiences with endometriosis. I found this was helpful in making sense of my own experience and in ensuring I could present the consultant with clear information to inform decision making. In situations where our appointments are often time-pressured, I also found this enables the consultant to quickly understand my history and focus on the presenting problem. It also made me feel more in control of a situation in which I frequently felt out of control and overwhelmed.

In chapter 8, we will cover how to be assertive in asking for what you need in more detail, but it is helpful to outline my appointment in relation to this timeline here. I found that it was helpful to me to go into appointments with a clear question in mind. In psychology, we often call this a helping question. In other words, what is the question I want help answering in this appointment? When I prepared this timeline, my question was what are my current treatment options, and would a hysterectomy be of any benefit to me as it was not a cure for endometriosis? If you have a clear idea of what you need to know from the appointment, then the consultant is more likely to be able to provide you with helpful information. I have attended endless appointments where I have felt I was not listened to, and I did not understand the information I was given or the reasons behind the recommendations that were made. I was often left feeling I had been given generic advice that I felt had been repeated to every person the consultant had seen that day. I have found

An Introduction to Me and My Journey

that approaching the appointment with a clear question and objective in mind can go some way towards preventing this.

Initial Background	Started periods when I was 12 – quickly progressed to very heavy periods causing significant pain.
	From the age of 14, I had repeated episodes of fainting, cystitis, and fatigue. I also developed ongoing lower back pain, leg pain, and cramps after my periods started. These symptoms were always attributed to other things, e.g. back pain attributed to being tall (I'm 5ft 11), leg pain attributed to 'lax ligaments', and fainting to low blood pressure/stress. I had one admission to the hospital connected with the pain and a UTI when I was around 13/14 years old. This was treated with IV antibiotics, pain relief, and I was sent home without any follow-up care.
	Mum took me to the GP multiple times – told it was dysmenorrhoea (painful, heavy periods) – prescribed the combined contraceptive pill at 15 which controlled my symptoms when taken without a break.
	At 20 years old, I developed migraines, and the combined pill was stopped. I started taking a 'mini pill' (progesterone only) instead, and I also tried a contraceptive injection as an alternative to the mini pill. Both treatments were only partially effective. I experienced lots of between cycle bleeding, an irregular cycle, and ongoing significant pain. I tried a contraceptive injection for around 9 months as the GP advised it would "take time to settle". After 9 months, I gave up and continued with the mini pill as although still only partially effective, it was better than the injection for me.
	Whilst taking the mini pill, I consistently experienced discomfort during sex, which increased over time. I also began to experience bleeding after sex in my late 20s which continued until my hysterectomy.
	Once I stopped the mini pill, I began to experience increasing urinary difficulties. This was generally treated as cystitis but then developed repeated UTIs. This was one of the first symptoms that became very difficult to manage, and I repeatedly sought medical help for.

(*Continued*)

(*Continued*)

October/November 2009	Repeated presentations to the GP with severe lower back pain and urinary symptoms. At one point, pelvic inflammatory disease was mentioned but not explained or explored.
	I continued to experience recurrent UTIs and cystitis. I was advised to use over-the-counter medication for the cystitis and was given antibiotics when needed for the UTIs.
	One of these infections caused me to become increasingly unwell and I presented at the GP multiple times. After being sent home the day before, I went back again and I collapsed in the GP surgery in significant pain and was subsequently admitted to hospital.
	I was diagnosed with a kidney infection (pyelonephritis). This infection became very serious, resulting in urosepsis which is a kind of sepsis caused by a urinary infection. This led to problems with my lungs (acute lung injury) – I was acutely unwell at this time and admitted to the high dependency unit (HDU).
	I was discharged from hospital in December 2009 and was under the care of urology post-discharge but also referred to gynaecology.
January–May 2010	Returned to work on a phased return. Ongoing difficulties with my lungs following the admission to HDU. Ongoing back pain and urinary difficulties.
	Ongoing tests between this and next appointment including CT scan. Prescribed long-term antibiotics on discharge from the hospital and advised to continue taking the mini pill. My recovery from this episode took approximately 18 months, and my gynaecological symptoms continued. I think that this admission caused confusion as the focus became on my kidneys, and I think this led to 'missing' the possible endometriosis.
October 2010	Met consultant 1 for an outpatient appointment – reported ongoing pain and fatigue as well as episodes of feeling unwell. I said this appeared worse around the time of my menstrual cycle and was advised to continue the antibiotics and mini pill.

(*Continued*)

(Continued)

2010–2012	Slow recovery from the kidney infection and associated complications. Continued antibiotics for 18 months in total. Ongoing difficulties with: • Severe left-sided pain • Back pain • Leg pain • Irregular menstrual cycle • Bleeding • Headaches • Fatigue • Discomfort during sex I had been discharged from outpatients but continued to present at the GP and was eventually re-referred to urology outpatients.
May 2012	Met consultant 2 for an outpatient appointment documenting painful periods (dysmenorrhoea) and previous kidney infection (acute pyelonephritis). The letter states I was presenting with recurrent left-sided pain and blood in the urine, as well as ongoing urinary difficulties (which I now believe were interstitial cystitis). I was reminded that recovery may be significant due to the severity of previous episode – plan to follow up in 5-6 months. No further action plan was recommended or documented in the letter.
September 2012	Another outpatient appointment with consultant 2 documenting the same symptoms and difficulties as in May 2012. No improvement in my symptoms, so consultant 2 suggested a renal biopsy, which I declined as I did not feel my symptoms were connected to my renal system. I was discharged back to GP on the basis that they could do nothing else for me.

(Continued)

(*Continued*)

2012 – 2015	Completed my doctorate in clinical psychology with ongoing symptoms managed as best I could at that time. Symptoms included: • Chronic pain, particularly on the left side • Leg pain • Heavy bleeding including clotting • Migraines • Bloating • Pain after sex • Bladder symptoms I continued to take the mini pill mainly for contraceptive purposes as I did not feel it was having any impact on my other symptoms. Stopped the pill at the end of 2014 as I wanted to conceive. Presented to the GP during this time due to discomfort during intercourse and after sex. No treatment plan given.
May 2015	Colposcopy for bleeding between periods and after sex – it was noted that some of the cells from inside my cervix were noticeable outside my cervix (cervical ectropion) and there was inflammation in this area. Cervical screen had shown some abnormal cells, so I had a biopsy which was normal and then I was discharged. Sometime later, I had the cervical ectropion burnt away (cauterised) by the GP to see if this would reduce the bleeding between periods and after sex. This did not make a significant difference to either symptom. Urinary symptoms persisted and in May 2015, I was admitted to hospital and treated for suspected UTI. I fell pregnant shortly after this. No significant difficulties with becoming pregnant.

(*Continued*)

An Introduction to Me and My Journey

(*Continued*)

May–December 2015	Pregnancy.
	I found pregnancy difficult. I experienced bleeding in first trimester and significant pain throughout. Diagnosed with pelvic girdle pain in second trimester – was unable to work from approx. 32 weeks. I was in considerable pain throughout my pregnancy, with early bleeding resulting in early scans. Later, I experienced increased monitoring due to concerns about the baby being too big, which involved consultant number 3.
	I was induced following my water breaking and had a vaginal birth at 38 weeks.
2016–2018	I had a hormonal coil fitted after giving birth as I was concerned about forgetting to take my pill. I did not want to try the contraceptive injection again, so the coil was suggested as an alternative. I had lots of difficulties with this from the point of insertion. I made repeated visits to the GP due to pain and bleeding – as with other forms of contraception in the past. I thought my difficulties in the first year of my daughter's life were due to recovery from a difficult pregnancy and previous difficulties with my health.
	In early 2017, my difficulties escalated. The GP suggested to continue with the coil as it can take time to settle. It had been in situ for approx. 12 months. I presented a couple of months later and had it removed.
	Symptoms then escalated further, culminating in hospital admission.

(*Continued*)

COPING WITH ENDOMETRIOSIS

(*Continued*)

March 2018	I had an admission to hospital early March 2018 – I was experiencing lots of pain in my abdomen and back. Due to my UTI history, I was treated for suspected UTI. I was referred to gynaecology but due to hospital pressures was not seen before discharge and was advised to ask my GP to be referred as an outpatient if the pain continued.
	Symptoms continued to worsen significantly on return home. I collapsed and was re-admitted via ambulance with suspected sepsis for the second time.
	I was seen by gynaecology (consultant number 4) and found I had a significant pelvic infection that had remained untreated – consultant 4 advised this could have been for as long as 12 months. I had surgery to remove the infection from the pelvis. My fallopian tubes were damaged by the infection. I was advised I may now have increased difficulties conceiving, and I would be be at high risk for ectopic pregnancy. If I became pregnant, I was to present to gynaecology for early scanning. This would be a permanent risk factor.
	Discharge document states laparoscopic drainage of pelvic abscess and pelvic washout. It also states I had been counselled on the risks of future pregnancies when I was merely advised of the risk factors. I asked about the possibility of endometriosis whilst in hospital but was advised by consultant 4 that my pelvis was 'in such a mess we wouldn't have been able to tell even if there was some there, until all the inflammation goes down'.
May–December 2018	I was seen in gynaecology outpatients by consultant number 5. My symptoms continued and were becoming increasingly severe over time. I was prescribed the mini pill again and when this did not control my symptoms, consultant 5 advised to double the dose. This caused significant bleeding and no improvement in functioning. I was told a laparoscopy would be 'pointless' because the likelihood was that I had 'something like endometriosis', but I could consider a hysterectomy. When I declined this, I was discharged.
	I was advised I could be re-referred to the same consultant but was extremely unhappy with the care I had received.

(*Continued*)

An Introduction to Me and My Journey

(*Continued*)

January–June 2019	I felt in need of a second opinion, and I was financially supported by my family to be able to access an appointment with consultant number 6 privately.

I wanted to explore options for laparoscopy, at this time I still did not have a confirmed diagnosis of endometriosis or any other condition.

Consultant 6 advised there was no need for a laparoscopy as my symptoms were clearly endometriosis related, and this could be treated as a 'clinical diagnosis' without investigation. He therefore suggested a 'radical hysterectomy' including opening my abdomen and removing my womb, cervix, fallopian tubes, and both ovaries. I asked if any other options were available, such as a laparoscopic hysterectomy or leaving my ovaries intact. However, consultant 6 recommended an 'all or nothing approach' and if I was going to have surgery it 'made sense to take the whole lot'.

He prescribed hormone blockers to 'shut down the system' placing me into menopause at 31 years old. His feeling was that this would allow me to assess whether a radical hysterectomy was the right option for me. I initially had hormone blockers without HRT which caused significant side effects. I began HRT, but some symptoms (including pain) continued. |
| June 2019 | Ongoing discomfort and pain. Prescribed antibiotics for presumed relapse of pelvic infection, although this was not confirmed on tests.

I discussed concerns about hormone blockers and HRT with consultant 6. I explained I did not want to continue with this and asked if there were other options to manage my symptoms. I still felt unsure about a radical hysterectomy and had been researching other treatment options available, which I was being told were not an option for me.

Consultant 6 suggested I go without any hormonal intervention so that I could see 'how bad it would be' and this would 'reassure' me about the need for hysterectomy. Consultant 6 continued to refuse laparoscopy surgery or the option to retain my ovaries and stated that radical hysterectomy was the best option. |

(*Continued*)

(*Continued*)

June–December 2019	I engaged with Endometriosis UK and other support groups due to concerns about the care I was receiving. I became aware of the need to be seen by a specialist centre and went back to the GP with ongoing symptoms and to request a referral to specialist centre. GP supported this referral.
January 2020	I was seen by specialist centre by consultant number 7 and offered laparoscopy with removal of endometriosis (excision surgery) if required. Although this felt like progress, I still felt my symptoms were not being fully believed or understood. I was advised by consultant 7 that I may need referral to a chronic pain centre. I was given the impression that even if I had endometriosis, my experience of pain was still beyond what they would expect. This made me feel like they thought I was exaggerating, or the pain was 'in my head'. I was treated again with antibiotics for suspected pelvic infection and then given amitriptyline for pain. I took this for 12 weeks before stopping due to side effects and no difference in pain. I was just really sedated. I was told it was a 12-month minimum waiting time for laparoscopy.
March–September 2020	The COVID pandemic hit. Waiting times for NHS treatment significantly increased, and gynaecology waiting times were the worst hit. My health continued to decline as I awaited treatment.
October 2020	Consultant number 8 reviews this timeline, and we agree on a treatment plan (see below)

I met consultant 8 in October 2020. At our first appointment, he reviewed this timeline, and I explained the recommendations from consultants 6 and 7 – one for radical hysterectomy and one for exploratory laparoscopy and treatment under the chronic pain clinic. Consultant 8 talked me through all the available treatment options and the pros and cons of each one. His opinion was that I was highly likely to have severe endometriosis but that I may also have a condition called adenomyosis, which I had not heard of before. Adenomyosis is a condition where the lining of the womb starts to grow into the muscle wall of the womb (NHS UK, 2023). It is a different condition from endometriosis, but some research suggests up to 90% of people with endometriosis also have adenomyosis (Kunz et al., 2005). Consultant 8 thought I might have both conditions. In answer to my question about the value of hysterectomy, he said this in part depended on whether I had adenomyosis as although hysterectomy is not a cure for endometriosis, it is a cure for adenomyosis as this is a condition of the uterus.

We agreed I would have an MRI scan, which would be unlikely to show any endometriosis but may show adenomyosis. I felt this would help inform my decision making. My MRI scan showed my uterus was enlarged, and there was thickening suggestive of adenomyosis. I had a further two appointments with consultant 8 before making my decision to have a laparoscopic hysterectomy but to retain my ovaries if possible.

I underwent a laparoscopic hysterectomy in February 2021. Although the hope had been to retain my ovaries, the left ovary had to be removed due to significant scarring and damage. My right ovary was retained which has prevented the onset of menopause. Significant excision of endometriosis was performed as endometriosis was found throughout the pelvis and on my bowel. I was alone throughout this hospital admission and surgery due to COVID restrictions which made a difficult experience even more challenging. Despite this, 24 hours after surgery, I was in less pain than I had been for years. I knew very quickly that I had made the right decision for me. It is from this position that I now write this book, retrospectively looking back on lots of uncertainty but from a place of things being better.

I do not think my decision will be right for everyone reading this book, and it was not an easy decision for me. I do believe, however, that developing knowledge of the condition and the treatment options allowed me to make a fully informed decision about surgery. I had undergone many treatments previously where I do not feel I was fully informed and where I may have made different choices had different information been provided to me. I think it is therefore essential that you approach your own appointments with a basic understanding of endometriosis and the associated conditions and misdiagnoses that come with it, so you can advocate for yourself and make the choices that feel right for you. This does require a degree of assertiveness, which can be difficult and a topic we will revisit in chapter 8.

Now I have introduced myself and my journey, I want to introduce you to endometriosis and the menstrual cycle, as understanding this has been essential for me to make sense of my difficulties. I then want to introduce you to Paul Gilbert's model of compassion-focused therapy. Chapters 2 and 3 then build the foundations for the rest of the book, so I would encourage you not to skip over these. Later in the book, you can be more flexible in picking which chapters you feel apply to you and your experience, but this first section is the foundations to build.

2 Understanding Menstrual Health and Endometriosis

The aim of this book is not to provide medical diagnosis or advice, as that is beyond my professional expertise. Despite the recognised challenges of accessing healthcare and obtaining a diagnosis, it is important that you do seek medical advice and support for the symptoms you are experiencing. In this chapter, I am going to outline my understanding of menstrual health as I feel that this is important to understanding your own experience, being able to advocate for yourself, and making sense of the psychological impact of menstruation and associated gynaecological conditions. It takes an average of eight years from the onset of symptoms to receiving a diagnosis of endometriosis (Endometriosis UK, 2022). This delay is thought to be due to a lack of understanding in women themselves and a lack of training and awareness in the medical profession (Ballard, Lowton and Wright, 2006). Like many of the women in this research, I believed my symptoms were normal, which was reinforced by GPs who were the first healthcare professionals I approached for support. I think improving understanding for everyone starts with menstrual health education. I do not blame the healthcare professionals who were unable to understand what I was experiencing or provide a diagnosis. However, I do think this lack of understanding impacted the compassion I received at times. Although knowing more about menstrual health and endometriosis would not have cured me of the condition, I wonder how my experience might have been different if healthcare professionals had been more able to recognise and diagnose endometriosis and if I had been able to recognise my symptoms and access support and treatment earlier.

What Is Menstrual Health?

When I was at school, we were taught about periods. The medical term for a period is menstruation which is when the body sheds blood and the lining of the uterus (NHS, 2023). In recent years, the term menstrual health has emerged across advocacy organisations, within policy and research. It was defined in 2021 by the Terminology Action Group of the Global Menstrual Collective (Hennegan et al., 2021). Their definition is:

> *Menstrual health is a state of complete physical, mental, and social well-being and not merely the absence of disease or infirmity, in relation to the menstrual cycle.*

The definition goes on to highlight the many actions involved with achieving good menstrual health across our lives including being able to:

- access accurate, timely, age-appropriate information about the menstrual cycle, menstruation, and changes experienced throughout the life course, as well as related self-care and hygiene practices.
- care for their bodies during menstruation such that their preferences, hygiene, comfort, privacy, and safety are supported. This includes accessing and using effective and affordable menstrual materials and having supportive facilities and services, including water, sanitation, and hygiene services, for washing the body and hands, changing menstrual materials, and cleaning and/or disposing of used materials.
- access timely diagnosis, treatment, and care for menstrual cycle-related discomforts and disorders, including access to appropriate health services and resources, pain relief, and strategies for self-care.
- experience a positive and respectful environment in relation to the menstrual cycle, free from stigma and psychological distress,

including the resources and support they need to confidently care for their bodies and make informed decisions about self-care throughout their menstrual cycle.
- decide whether and how to participate in all spheres of life, including civil, cultural, economic, social, and political, during all phases of the menstrual cycle, free from menstrual-related exclusion, restriction, discrimination, coercion, and/or violence.

When I first read this definition, it reminded me how few of these points were met in my life. From my first lesson on periods, I lacked the information I needed to understand what menstrual health was, how to identify problems with my menstrual health, and how to access treatment and care. Not understanding menstrual health made it more taboo and meant I did not understand my experience was not 'normal' for a very long time. This meant that rather than knowing I needed help and support, I came to believe that I was coping badly with a normal period. This impacted on how I saw myself and my relationships with other people (see chapters 7, 8, and 9).

Menstrual health education is the foundation on which women and menstruating people can learn to understand and manage their cycle. In 2020, the UK government made it compulsory that menstrual well-being is taught in schools (Endometriosis, UK). This guidance states that all pupils regardless of their sex will be taught about menstrual well-being. It is hoped that this will reduce period stigma by promoting an inclusive approach to education (Rios, 2019).

This is very different to my own experience of menstrual education. I was educated in the 1990s – a time when conversations about sex, relationships, and periods were medical and focussed on reproduction. Most of my menstrual education came from my mum who was open, honest, and supportive throughout my endometriosis journey. However, the ability to discuss my experience with people other than my mum was hindered by the fact this was not something that anyone talked about, and I believe my menstrual health education did not provide me with the tools I needed to manage the difficulties I went on to face.

I was formally taught about periods for the first time at primary school. This was a one-off lesson in year six (age 10–11) where boys and girls were separated for sex education lessons. This meant the first time periods were discussed outside of my family, it was done in an all-female environment. We were explicitly told this was not for discussion with the boys in the class which introduced a message that periods were something shameful to be kept private. If you did need to talk about periods, you would ideally talk to another woman. I have struggled over the years to talk to other people, particularly men, about my periods and the problems they have caused. I think this has been another factor which has hindered my journey to a diagnosis as it prevented me from speaking openly about my symptoms. I also think this sets the scene for some of the shame I experienced later in life, as my overwhelming experience of medical care, particularly gynaecology, is that I have usually been speaking with a man. In 2021, most registered doctors in the UK were men. Although female GPs outnumbered their male counterparts, there was a pronounced gender gap among specialist doctors with more men than women in this profession, which would include gynaecology (data from Michas, 2022). In chapters 3 and 9, we will look at ways of talking about your difficulties to medical professionals, and I found this helpful when attending these appointments.

My menstrual education consisted of being taught what a period was, how it related to reproduction, and a limited amount of information on female hygiene products. We were told about period pains but that these were mild, manageable, and crucially were not an excuse not to do PE. I don't remember being told that periods can be different and not all periods are normal. There was no discussion about what you might worry about or need to see a doctor for. On reflection, I feel that it was this detail that could have made a difference to me understanding the initial signs something was not right with my menstrual health. For example, I was aware I would bleed, but not that this could be different amounts and some bleeding would be deemed heavy which was a reason to seek medical advice.

Unfortunately, my experience of menstrual education appears to be mirrored by other people in the UK. In 2018, Plan International UK reported that one in seven girls in the UK did not know what was happening when they started their periods, and a quarter did not know what to do (Promoting Menstrual Well-being, RCN). In 2021, the Department of Health found only 8% of women felt they had enough information about gynaecological conditions and 84% recalled incidents where they felt they had not been listened to by healthcare professionals. In 2022, Menstrual Health information was the most selected topic in the Women's Health Strategy for England survey for women aged 18–29 (DHSE, 2022).

My personal experience of menstrual education gave me three key messages:

1. Periods were a manageable part of life, and any discomfort could and should be tolerated. A period should not stop you from doing any of your normal activities, and if it did, you were using it as an excuse.
2. Talking about periods should be avoided. If you must talk about periods, you should try to talk to a woman if you can.
3. Periods are a normal part of life, and you should be able to manage them. Failure to cope with periods and their symptoms was attributable to you personally (e.g. 'having a low pain threshold').

I started my periods when I was 12 years old. Unlike some girls surveyed by Plan International UK, I did know what was happening and what to do (thanks mum). I wasn't distressed by my period starting and remember feeling a sense of relief that this long-anticipated thing had finally happened. I had no awareness that my life would change drastically following the onset of my menstrual cycle. Within a year, I had my first hospital admission connected with 'problem periods'. It then took a further 20 years to gain a full understanding of my periods and that they were not simply a problem, nor was I the problem. I was dealing with a medically diagnosable long-term, incurable condition.

The Menstrual Cycle: Medical Phases and Changing Seasons

If your experience of menstrual education was like mine, you may still be trying to understand how your menstrual cycle works. For me, I didn't understand that you are always in your menstrual cycle, and this can be impacting you in different ways at different times. Understanding the menstrual cycle as a whole and how this impacted me helped me to make sense of my symptoms and explain them more coherently to medical professionals. For this reason, I am going to share my understanding of the menstrual cycle here and how I came to understand this for myself from resources I accessed during my journey.

The onset of menstruation is a physical and psychological milestone in the life of a menstruating person (RCN, 2022). The NHS online (2022a) provides an overview of the menstrual cycle and the three phases that occur in the ovaries and walls of the uterus in response to the rise and fall of different hormone levels. This is a summary of that information which you can also access via their website (see reference list). A menstrual cycle can vary from 23 to 35 days. Different phases of the cycle can impact you in different ways, and you may experience different symptoms at different times.

> Phase 1: The Menstrual Phase. The word 'period' generally refers to the menstrual phase of the cycle, which is when you experience a bleed. This bleed can last between two and seven days with varying menstrual flow. The first day you bleed is the first day of your menstrual cycle (helpful for tracking). Periods lasting

more than seven days are one reason to speak to a healthcare professional.

Phase 2: The Follicular Phase: This phase of the menstrual cycle is preparing for ovulation. At this time, follicle-stimulating hormone (FSH) is produced to stimulate egg development. This will result in the maturation and release of an egg, known as ovulation. This phase starts on the first day of your period and lasts for 13–14 days, ending with ovulation.

Phase 3: Ovulation and the Luteal Phase: This phase (lasting 14 days) follows ovulation, which is where the egg travels and prepares for implantation. This can be a time you might experience some pre-menstrual symptoms such as aches, tender breasts, bloating, tiredness, and mood changes.

I had an understanding of my period from my early teens, but I found it very difficult to understand why I experienced so many symptoms at different times of the month which seemed disconnected to my period. I think this was because I did not understand that there are phases to the menstrual cycle, and in each phase something is happening in the female body connected with menstruation. No one ever made it clear to me that even though you are not constantly having a period, you are constantly within the menstrual cycle. All these changes can impact you in different ways, and so all parts of the cycle, not just the period, could be relevant to you and your experience.

The most helpful way I found to understand this was the idea that you can think about your menstrual cycle like the seasons of the year (Hill, 2019). Both are cyclical, and they keep moving, sometimes you don't notice the season and sometimes it's the focus of your day. Sometimes, you will change your plans along with the season. I found this a useful way to think about how to manage my experience in different menstrual 'seasons' (phases). Although I first read this idea in Maisie Hill's book, I have since seen it presented elsewhere and have chosen to present my version of this idea here in the hope it is also helpful for you.

Winter (the menstrual phase)	Spring (the follicular phase)
In winter, when you are on your period, you might feel like hiding away from the world. Your hormone levels are at their lowest and you might feel more tired than usual, in pain or experiencing other symptoms. You might also be craving certain foods along with warmth and other comfort. This was a hard phase for me, and I would often be in a lot of pain. I did feel like I wanted to curl up in a ball somewhere, away from others, until it was over.	Your period has ended! You might feel more refreshed and relieved – a boost of oestrogen may make you feel more energised at this time. You might feel freer and brighter than you did in the winter. I did used to feel relief when my period was over, as the management of multiple symptoms all at once reduced.
Summer (the ovulatory phase)	Autumn (the luteal phase)
Your oestrogen levels are at their highest so you might be building on the tasks of the spring, feeling ready to socialise or focus on your goals. In the early phases of the disease, I did feel more positive in the spring and summer, but in the later stages of my condition, there was struggle associated with all the seasons.	Autumn weather is constantly changing, and the days start to get shorter and darker. It can be a tricky time of year to transition to darker nights, and this can feel the same for your menstrual cycle. This might be the phase you experience pre-menstrual symptoms including mood swings, skin breakouts, irritability, and bloating. I suffered with migraines in the autumn, a symptom I still experience in line with my ovulation cycle, although I no longer have a period.

Although I find this a helpful way to summarise and understand the menstrual cycle, it is worth noting that we are still speaking about a typical menstrual cycle. If you are reading this book, chances are this is not your experience. As an example, I found my summer was equally as difficult as winter. I noticed that the increased levels of oestrogen were linked to several symptoms for me, particularly debilitating pain and migraine. Although I no longer have a period, I have an ovary, and I continue to have a cycle because of this linked to ovulation. I still track this cycle as a way of understanding what is going on in my body at different times of the month. I still have an autumn and a winter phase where I am more fatigued, irritable, and emotional. I also have some of my past pain symptoms return including migraine and leg pain. I would encourage you to notice what the seasons are like for you – it isn't the same for all of us.

Menstrual Tracking

One of the hardest things in my journey was knowing what was 'normal'. As discussed above, there is a medical expectation for a normal menstrual cycle, but there are variations from person to person. With any bodily experience, you can only know what this experience is like for you, and it is important to have a sense of your own cycle so you can identify patterns and challenges. Also, if you do need medical intervention and treatment, it can be helpful to present your cycle alongside your timeline. This can aid decision making in terms of diagnosis and treatment.

I found it helpful to track my menstrual cycle and my wider symptoms so I could understand what was happening in my body. My endometriosis resulted in a wide range of difficulties, and it took me years to realise that they were symptoms of the disease and linked to my menstrual cycle. If you are reading this trying to work out whether your experiences are also symptoms, I would suggest tracking your symptoms as well as your menstrual cycle as you will then become aware if the symptoms are following a pattern and therefore might be linked. You can also use the symptoms section of this book to see if your experiences could be a symptom of endometriosis.

Retaining an ovary means I still have symptoms which follow a cyclical pattern in line with my previous menstrual cycle. However, these symptoms have significantly reduced since the surgery. The main ones that remain are fatigue, feeling more emotionally vulnerable, migraines (approximately once a month), and leg/hip pain – all occurring in a seven- to ten-day block. I have personally found that understanding your cycle can help with predicting when symptoms may arise and be problematic for you which means you may be able to adjust your life accordingly. I also find it easier to stay out of tricky loops (see chapter 3) and manage any anxiety related to symptoms if I know why they are occurring. For example, if I experience pain, I can link it to ovulation which prevents me from overthinking it or viewing the pain as a sign of endometriosis returning or worsening again. For me, the early stages of the disease had parts of the month that were worse and parts that were better so getting an understanding of this was very helpful. However, in the latter stages of the disease, my symptoms were more chronic, so the tracking focused on collating my symptoms with a view to making decisions on my treatment options. Like the timeline presented in chapter 1, my cycle tracking was something I was able to share with my consultant to inform my treatment planning. If you are in the early stages of your journey, your cycle tracking may be the first evidence you have accumulated on your difficulties to share with medical professionals.

There are many period trackers available including apps on your phone. I am not recommending any specific option but encouraging you to look at those available and see what works for you. Some of these are free and some offer a subscription service. However, you can do this yourself with a pen and paper. I used a paper version at first as this was easier for me to take along to my doctor's appointments and show to them. I also kept a file of my medical documents as I saw multiple professionals, and they would not always have access to the same notes or systems. If you want to use a paper tracker, I have included a table below. I would suggest listing your main symptoms and then giving them a code (either an abbreviation or a colour) so you can quickly fill the table out. You may also want to add your 'seasons' to think about what is helpful for you during those times, for example hibernation in winter. You could colour the background to represent this.

When I was tracking my symptoms, I did not do this more than once a day. If I missed some days, chances are they had been slightly better so I might leave those blank and just input when I had symptoms (or experiences I thought were symptoms). I initially tracked things I thought were symptoms, but as I learnt more about endometriosis, I realised that there were other parts of my experience that could be related to endometriosis, and I did not know that. You may want to look at the list of symptoms later in this book and use this to guide you on what to track from your own cycle.

Understanding Menstrual Health and Endometriosis

	Jan	Feb	Mar	April	May	June	July	Aug	Sept	Oct	Nov	Dec
1												
2												
3												
4												
5												
6												
7												
8												
9												
10												
11												
12												
13												
14												
15												
16												
17												
18												
19												
20												
21												
22												
23												
24												
25												
26												
27												
28												
29												
30												
31												

Symptom	Code	Notes

Season	Symptoms	Things I need in this season (these might be things you need to do or things you need to avoid)
Winter (the period/bleed)		
Spring		
Summer		
Autumn		

Endometriosis and Other Gynaecological Conditions

I did not hear the word endometriosis until ten years after my periods started. It was another ten years before I received a formal diagnosis. In addition to endometriosis, my MRI was suggestive of adenomyosis. Endometriosis is becoming more widely discussed and recognised than it was, but data from Endometriosis UK (2020) shows that 54% of people do not know what endometriosis is, increasing to 74% of men. Even when I heard the term endometriosis and I began trying to learn more about it, it was years before I felt I had a reasonable understanding of the condition. You may be pre-diagnosis, or post-diagnosis, but wherever you are in your journey I think it is useful to highlight what endometriosis is as well as some of the other gynaecological conditions that can occur.

What Is Endometriosis?

The NHS defines endometriosis as a condition where tissue like the lining of the womb starts to grow in other places, such as the ovaries and fallopian tubes (NHS, 2022b). I initially understood endometriosis to be the womb lining being in other places in the body, but this is incorrect as it is not the womb lining itself, but similar cells reacting the same way as tissues in the womb, building up and then breaking down and bleeding (Endometriosis UK, 2023). Unlike the cells in the womb that leave the body as a period, these cells elsewhere in the body have nowhere to escape. This can cause inflammation, pain, and the formation of scar tissue.

Like the cells inside the womb, these similar cells respond to the hormonal changes associated with the menstrual cycle and therefore endometriosis symptoms are often cyclical (which is why it is worth understanding and tracking your whole cycle). I think the fact that symptoms can come and go in line with your cycle is a factor that makes diagnosis difficult, as you may not link symptoms together (see list of symptoms later in this chapter). I did not link some of my symptoms together until I met with the surgeon who did my hysterectomy (consultant 8 in my timeline). Many of the symptoms of endometriosis may not be obvious as 'period related', and I think this contributes to the delay in diagnosis. For example, the migraine I get alongside ovulation was attributed to stress for years!

Endometriosis: Prevalence, Signs, Symptoms, and Classification

In the UK, around 1.5 million women and those assigned female at birth are currently living with endometriosis, regardless of race or ethnicity (Endometriosis UK, 2023). In 2010, the prevalence was estimated at 1.7 billion women worldwide (Adamson, Kennedy and

Hummelshoj, 2010). There is currently no cure for endometriosis, and it can have a significant impact on your daily life. For others, the impact of having endometriosis may be smaller. Some people with endometriosis may have no symptoms at all. This means it is possible that there are many more people living with endometriosis than the figures suggest.

There are several symptoms of endometriosis outlined by the NHS. Not everyone with endometriosis will experience all of these, and this is not an exhaustive list. However, symptoms can include:

- pain in your lower tummy or back (pelvic pain) – usually worse during your period
- period pain that stops you from doing your normal activities
- pain during or after sex
- pain when peeing or pooing during your period
- feeling sick, constipation, diarrhoea, or blood in your pee during your period
- difficulty getting pregnant
- heavy periods.

There are many subcategories to these symptoms and other symptoms that have been reported. Endometriosis UK (2023) summarises these as follows:

Pain symptoms	Bleeding symptoms	Bowel and bladder symptoms	Other symptoms
Painful periods	Prolonged bleeding	Painful bowel movements	Tiredness/lack of energy/fatigue
Pain on ovulation	'Spotting' or bleeding between periods	Bleeding from the bowel	Depression/anxiety
Pain during an internal examination for example a smear test	Heavy bleeding with or without clots	Symptoms of irritable bowel (diarrhoea, constipation, bloating – particularly during your period)	

(Continued)

(Continued)

Pain symptoms	Bleeding symptoms	Bowel and bladder symptoms	Other symptoms
Pain during or after sex (intercourse/penetration and/or orgasm)	Loss of 'old' or 'dark blood' before period	Pain when passing urine	Relationship difficulties including sex life
Pelvic pain		Pain before or after passing urine or opening bowel	Difficulties with activities of daily living/maintaining occupation
Chronic/persistent pain			

In my experience, the initial symptoms of endometriosis were transient (cyclical) and therefore easier to manage. I did have a spring/summer that was significantly better than autumn/winter so it made it easier to take time to rest in the winter, knowing that spring was coming and there would be respite again. However, as time progressed, I became increasingly impacted by the condition to the point where my quality of life was significantly impaired, and I felt like I was living in Narnia – stuck in an eternal winter. I found this difficult to talk to others about, and I feel that made many things more difficult, particularly my work.

When my condition was at its worst, I needed support with several things in my daily life. It became increasingly apparent I could no longer function as an able-bodied individual. I tried for a long time to ignore this fact and carry on regardless to my own detriment. I was forced to confront the reality of my condition on a family holiday to Disneyland Paris. I had been prepared that this trip would be difficult as my functioning was poor at that stage due to persistent, often debilitating pain and other symptoms. For the first time in my life, I had admitted my limitations and accessed the GP for a letter of support to get an access pass at Disneyland as I knew I would not be able to queue for long periods of time. I was determined that the trip would not be impacted by my condition and my daughter would not miss out. I believed that I would be able to manage the trip. Despite making multiple adaptations, by the end of the first day I could barely walk due to the pain and needed a wheelchair for the following days. This was a steep learning curve for me as I felt forced to recognise that I was now disabled by my illness. This was something I found difficult to accept and factored into my later decision to have a hysterectomy.

Endometriosis itself is not a disability, which is the same as other long-term conditions which are covered in the Equality Act 2010. You may be defined as disabled under the Equality Act 2010 if you have 'a physical or mental impairment that has a "substantial" and "long-term" negative effect on your ability to do normal daily activities'. An example of substantial might be that it takes you much longer to complete a daily task, such as getting dressed, than it would be for another person without an impairment. Long term is defined as lasting for 12 months or more. If you are disabled by your endometriosis, its symptoms, or other factors associated with the impact of the disease you may be able to access support with employment or be eligible for financial support if you are unable to work. More information on this can be found online via the Department for Work and Pensions website.

Endometriosis Classification

When I began using online forums for support, I noticed lots of people talking about what stage of endometriosis they had. The stages of endometriosis were not covered on the NHS website, so I did not understand what they referred to. I was left feeling confused. I then read the NICE guidance (2017) for the diagnosis and management of endometriosis, which states that endometriosis should be managed according to the severity of the symptoms rather than the stage of the disease. This means in the UK, many medical professionals are moving away from classifying endometriosis according to stages. However, some still do, and I was given a stage for my endometriosis by my consultant (stage 4).

If you are using online forums or social media to inform your understanding of your condition, I think it is helpful to understand that there is a staging system for classifying endometriosis although this is no longer recommended by NICE in the UK. If you live outside of the UK, this system may still be in place. NICE guidance in the UK suggests staging systems should not be used; however, the World Endometriosis Society (Johnson et al., 2017) suggests that all women must complete the American Society of Reproductive Medicine (ASRM) classification until a better system becomes available. This is a summary of what I understand about the staging system for endometriosis. In 1979, the ASRM came up with four stages of endometriosis which were designed to classify the severity of the disease, from mild to severe. This system was revised in 1984. However, the classification systems that have been used in the past have all been criticised for sharing the same weakness – a poor correlation between the classification given and the symptoms experienced (Soo-Young, Koo, and Dae-Hyung, 2021). This means that your endometriosis can be classified as stage 1, but you might be significantly impacted by your symptoms or stage 4 with little impact on your life. This can be invalidating for people living with endometriosis.

For many years, I struggled to get a diagnosis and was left feeling that I must, therefore, only be at a mild stage of the disease. This confirmed what I had already begun to believe at that time – that this wasn't a big thing, and I was coping badly with a mild problem. When I had my surgery, I was told that my endometriosis was stage 4 and had begun to infiltrate my bowel. I was shown the pictures from my surgery at my request, and I felt relieved that I could see the endometriosis on the images. There was also a part of me that wanted to be told it was severe to validate my pain and my journey. I was afraid that if it wasn't severe, this would confirm the messages I had received for years that I was making a big deal out of nothing.

I cannot say it to my younger self, but I can say to you that the stage of your endometriosis does not relate to your symptoms or your experience. Your experience is valid – you are not making it up or exaggerating. You do not have to be in stage 3 or 4 to be suffering. If you are suffering, that is enough for you to be treated with compassion and respect. This is not in your head, and you are not alone. You are dealing with something that not even the medical professionals can agree on how to classify yet.

Other Gynaecological Conditions

This book focuses on endometriosis, but there are many other gynaecological conditions that can co-exist with endometriosis or by themselves. You will notice that there are many overlaps with the symptoms of endometriosis presented above, so it is important to see a GP if you are experiencing any gynaecological symptoms to ensure you are receiving the right treatment. I think the overlaps are one of the many complexities of diagnosing and receiving support for endometriosis.

This list of gynaecological conditions is taken from NICE (2017), and the symptoms are taken from the NHS website which you can access. I have added Adenomyosis as this was my co-morbid diagnosis.

Cervical Cancer: Cancer that is found anywhere in the cervix, which is the opening between the vagina and the womb (uterus). Nearly all cervical cancers are caused by an infection from certain types of human papillomavirus (HPV). Cervical screening (smear tests) checks for changes to cervical cells with a view to identify the cause for any changes and determine appropriate treatment pathways. Symptoms include vaginal bleeding that is unusual for you such as bleeding after sex, changes to vaginal discharge, pain during sex, and pain in your low back, pelvis, or lower tummy.

Polycystic Ovary Syndrome (PCOS): PCOS is a common condition thought to affect one in ten women in the UK. It impacts how the ovaries work, and they become enlarged and contain fluid-filled sacs which surround the eggs. These sacs mean that ovulation might not always take place which can cause difficulty getting pregnant. The main symptoms are irregular periods, excess androgen (hormones which can cause excess facial or body hair), weight gain, thinning hair/hair loss, and acne.

Fibroids: Fibroids are non-cancerous growths that develop in or around the womb. They are made up of muscle and fibrous tissue. Many women are unaware that they have fibroids as they do not cause any symptoms, but fibroids are sometimes identified by changes during routine gynaecological examinations, tests, or scans. When symptoms are present, they can include heavy or painful periods, abdominal pain, lower back pain, frequent need to urinate, constipation, and pain or discomfort during sex.

Heavy Menstrual Bleeding (menorrhagia): You are expected to lose 4–12 teaspoons of blood in a normal period, with two heavy days which then become lighter. A heavy period may require changing a pad or tampon more often, for example, every one to two hours. When using a menstrual cup, you may need to empty it more frequently. You may also need to use two types of sanitary products together, such as a pad and a tampon. You may also bleed through your clothes or bedding and may pass clots larger than a 10p coin. The NHS website has a self-assessment tool you can use to establish whether you are experiencing heavy periods. This can be accessed via their website.

Ovarian Cancer: Ovarian cancer affects the ovaries and mostly affects people over the age of 50. The symptoms are not always obvious, and it can run in families. Symptoms of ovarian cancer include a swollen tummy/bloating; pain in the pelvis, no appetite or feeling full quickly after eating, needing to urinate more often, indigestion, bowel problems, back pain, fatigue, and weight loss.

Pelvic Organ Prolapse: Pelvic organ prolapse is when one or more of the organs in the pelvis slip down from their normal position and bulge into the vagina. This can cause pain and discomfort. Symptoms include a feeling of heaviness in your lower tummy and genitals, a dragging discomfort in your vagina, feeling like there is something coming down into your vagina, feeling or seeing a bulge or lump in or coming out of your vagina, discomfort during sex, and problems urinating. There are several things that increase your risk of organ prolapse including pregnancy and childbirth, menopause, being overweight, long-term constipation, and hysterectomy.

Pelvic Inflammatory Disease (PID): PID is an infection of the female reproductive system including the womb, fallopian tubes, and ovaries. Sometimes, PID does not cause any symptoms. It can cause mild symptoms (which overlap with other conditions) including pelvic pain, pain during sex, pain when urinating, bleeding between periods and after sex, heavy/painful periods, and unusual vaginal discharge. A few people (me included) become very unwell with PID – these symptoms include severe pain in the tummy/pelvis, a high temperature, and feeling/being sick. The NHS website states that most cases of PID are caused by a bacterial infection that is spread from the vagina or cervix to the organs which are higher up. In many cases it is caused by a sexually transmitted infection – however, this is not the only cause. When I had PID (that resulted in sepsis and surgery), it was initially misdiagnosed as a UTI. It was later discovered that I most likely developed an infection connected with inserting or removing the coil. I would encourage you to access regular sexual health screening as part of caring for your menstrual health and wellbeing but also to be aware that a STI is not the only cause of PID.

Adenomyosis: Adenomyosis is a condition where the lining of the womb (endometrium) is found deep in the muscle of the uterus (myometrium). It is estimated to affect one in ten women of reproductive age and is more common in women aged 40–50 who have had children. The most common symptoms include heavy, painful, or irregular periods, pre-menstrual pelvic pain, and feelings of heaviness or discomfort in the pelvis. There is an association between adenomyosis and endometriosis. In 2015, Leyendecker et al. reported that 91.1% of women with adenomyosis in their study also had endometriosis.

Endometriosis Treatments

Currently there is no cure for endometriosis, but there are a range of treatments available that all aim to reduce the severity of the symptoms. If symptoms of endometriosis are well managed, this can have a positive impact on quality of life. In the early part of my journey (before I was around 23 years old) my symptoms were well controlled by taking hormonal contraceptives, and this meant endometriosis had very little impact on my quality of life. This book does not set out to discuss the pros and cons of different treatments or give any recommendations. Different treatments are suitable for different people – you may also try different treatments at different times in your journey (I have tried most of the treatments presented here). However, I do think it is useful to provide a summary of the current options available. All decisions about treatment need to be made based on individual guidance from a medical professional who can advise on the options available to you and help you to make informed choices. This is adapted from the information available from Endometriosis UK, NHS website, and NICE guidance for endometriosis (see reference list).

Hormonal Treatments: Endometriosis responds to the hormone oestrogen, so hormonal treatments aim to block or reduce the production of oestrogen in the body. This aims to stop the endometriosis growing and relieve symptoms. Examples of hormonal treatments include the combined contraceptive pill (the pill), progesterones (mini pill and contraceptive injection), and GnRH analogues which block oestrogen placing the body in temporary menopause.

Surgical Treatments: There are three types of surgery for endometriosis. Conservative surgery, usually done via laparoscopy, aims to remove or destroy the endometriosis. This can be done using excision surgery, where the endometriosis is cut out, or ablation where the endometriosis is destroyed using heat or laser. Complex surgery is when there are multiple organs affected by the endometriosis so more than one specialist may need to be involved in the operation. Radical surgery is considered where other treatment options have not been effective or suitable and the person is not looking to have children. Radical surgery mainly refers to a hysterectomy (removal of the womb) and/or oophorectomy (removal of the ovaries). Some people will have both the womb and their ovaries removed at the same time – others may have something different. In my case, I had my womb, cervix, fallopian tubes, and one ovary removed, as well as an excision of endometriosis throughout my pelvis and on my bowel.

All these treatments have advantages and disadvantages and must be considered on an individual basis with the support of a healthcare professional. In chapters 8 and 10 we will consider how to advocate for yourself and make decisions about treatment in more detail.

Summary

- Menstrual health refers to a complete sense of well-being in relation to the menstrual cycle, including understanding it and knowing how to manage it. It also includes being able to seek and access support and help if needed.
- The menstrual cycle extends beyond the period. Different phases of the menstrual cycle can impact us in different ways, and it can be helpful to understand what this looks like for you as a way of managing your menstrual health.
- Menstrual tracking can be a helpful tool to understand your cycle and to make links between your cycle and the symptoms you are experiencing. This can also be used as a tool to inform your diagnosis.
- Endometriosis has several symptoms which can overlap with other gynaecological conditions. It is important to understand your symptoms to inform treatment planning and symptom management.
- When seeking a diagnosis, it can help to be aware of and discuss other gynaecological conditions with a healthcare professional to ensure you are receiving the right treatment for you and your condition.
- There is currently no cure for endometriosis, but there are different treatments available to reduce the severity of the symptoms. Different treatments are suitable for different people, and all have pros and cons. All decisions about treatment need to be discussed with the medical professionals overseeing your care so you can make an informed decision about what is right for you.

3 A Psychological Understanding of Endometriosis Using Compassion-Focussed Therapy (CFT)

Psychological Thinking and Formulation

One of the fundamental aspects of psychological therapy is formulation. A psychological formulation usually uses a structured approach (meaning it follows a framework or model) that aims to understand the factors which contribute to the problem or distress we are experiencing. It aims to enable us to make sense of our experience so that we can begin to consider the changes needed to manage, or even overcome, our challenges.

For most of my journey, I was managing a collection of symptoms that I did not understand. Although endometriosis was mentioned at different points in my care, I did not receive that formal diagnosis until 20 years after I first presented with symptoms. I was told by several healthcare professionals that 'I probably had endometriosis', but I was not offered a laparoscopy in the earlier stages of my disease which is used to formally diagnose endometriosis. Although I was offered this when I accessed an endometriosis specialist centre by consultant number 8, by this time, I strongly believed that I had endometriosis. When my MRI results indicated I also had adenomyosis, I chose to have one surgery which would include both excision surgery if endometriosis was present and hysterectomy. This meant I never had a diagnostic laparoscopy to confirm my diagnosis, which was confirmed during my hysterectomy and excision surgery. It was terrifying going into that surgery not knowing if endometriosis would be found, and I doubted whether my symptoms were real right up until I saw the photos of my surgery. Prior to this, all I knew for sure was that I was managing a range of increasingly debilitating symptoms, and I was dealing with my emotional distress, much of which was driven by the impact the symptoms had on my quality of life and identity.

Usually when someone comes to see a clinical psychologist, they are experiencing some form of distress. This distress can present in lots of ways – it looks different for different people, and it looks different for the same person at different points in time. For me, my distress manifested in many ways over the years. I experienced hopelessness, fear, anxiety, anger, and shame. For some people, they may experience a mental health difficulty such as depression. Research has shown that 87% of women with endometriosis experience symptoms of depression and anxiety (Facchin et al., 2017). If you are experiencing symptoms of anxiety or depression, you may benefit from seeking further support with your mental health. I have summarised the symptoms of depression and anxiety here, so you can consider whether these might apply to you. Depression can impact the way we think and feel, the way we behave, and the way we interact with other people (NHS website, 2022). Not everyone with depression will experience the same symptoms, but these are some of the symptoms you might experience:

- Persistent low mood. You might feel sad or hopeless. You might be more tearful than usual.
- Low self-esteem.
- Lacking motivation to do things, or not enjoying the things you are doing as much as you usually would. Some people describe this as feeling like they are going through the motions.
- Being more impatient with other people and/or more irritable with them. You might avoid being around other people and withdraw from them.
- Finding it difficult to make decisions.

- Moving or speaking more slowly than usual.
- Changes in appetite (you may be eating more than usual or eating less). This might result in changes to your health or weight.
- Lack of energy.
- Sleep changes or problems. This might be sleeping more than usual, finding it difficult to get to sleep or waking frequently. You may also find that you do not feel rested, however much you sleep.
- Feeling that you do not want to live anymore, having thoughts of harming yourself or of ending your life. If this symptom applies to you, it is important you access support. All information on the support available in the UK can be found in chapter 10.

Anxiety can overlap with other mental health conditions such as generalised anxiety disorder, health anxiety, and obsessive compulsive disorder. Anxiety is a natural response to feelings of threat (see chapter 5) which we will all experience. However, sometimes anxiety can become persistent and have an impact on our daily life. This might be a time to seek professional support for anxiety. Like depression, anxiety can impact the way we think, behave, and interact with other people. Symptoms of anxiety can include:·

- Being more tired or restless than usual.
- Being irritable or short-tempered with others.
- Difficulties falling asleep or staying asleep.
- People who experience anxiety often report finding it difficult to get their brain to switch off or quieten down at night. They sometimes report waking up feeling anxiety in their body, but not knowing why.
- Physical symptoms such as being shaky, dizzy, and sweaty.
- People sometimes get headaches, migraines, tummy aches, or muscle pain linked to anxiety.

- Some people noticed a dry mouth or changes to their heart rate when anxious.
- Going over and over thoughts in their mind. This might be about the past or the future. Sometimes people worry about things that have happened that have caused them distress, or things that might happen. Sometimes it is a worry that 'something bad will happen', and this might be something that threatens their life or the life of people they care about, for example, worrying that a loved one will be involved in an accident every time they go out in the car.

There are several treatments available for anxiety and depression, including medication and psychological therapy. You can find information about anxiety, depression, and endometriosis from Endometriosis UK and MIND. There are resources available from the Compassionate Mind Foundation to think about compassionate approaches to these difficulties. Information about these can be found on their website. If you do need further support with these difficulties, I would encourage you to turn to chapter 10 where you will find information about the support available in the UK. Outside of the UK, I would recommend you speak to a healthcare professional for further advice.

Although I have never had a mental health diagnosis, I have had to work hard to manage the impact of endometriosis on my mental health. Over time, I have been able to use the skills I have learnt professionally to make sense of my own experience and learn different ways to manage my emotions. I think that without the ability to ask myself 'what would I say to a patient who was feeling this way?', I probably would have needed more support for my own mental health from professionals. Unfortunately, psychological support for the impact of living with endometriosis on my mental health and well-being was not available to me on the NHS where I live. I have accessed psychological therapy as a patient on more than one occasion in my life through different treatment avenues, as despite my professional knowledge there are times that I have needed more treatment and support than I could provide for myself. I accessed one of these courses of therapy privately, which I understand is not an option for everyone. If you are thinking about accessing therapy privately, you will find information in chapter 10 on how to find an accredited therapist or psychologist. However, I was able to access two of these services without a fee. One was through university as a student and one as an employee. I would encourage you to explore avenues for therapy in your educational and work settings as well as the NHS if this is something you feel would be helpful to you. However, therapy may not be available to everyone, and being able to share psychological ideas with those who are not able to access therapy is one of my hopes for this book.

In this chapter, I will share with you Paul Gilbert's model of compassion-focussed therapy (CFT). This is the model I have found most helpful to understand my own experience, and I hope it might be helpful for you to develop a psychological understanding of yours. I will also think about some of the factors that made it difficult for me to gain an understanding of what was happening to me. Throughout my journey, I lacked understanding. I did not understand what I was experiencing or how to manage it. I did not understand the impact it was having on my life and my identity. When I sought support to understand what was happening medically, it seemed medical professionals could not give me an understanding either, as they did not seem to understand themselves. People close to me found it difficult to understand my experience and over time, I stopped talking about it. I had begun to believe that I was the problem. Rather than understanding that I had a condition that needed treatment and help, I became ashamed and self-blaming. I believed I wasn't coping well with the pain, was eating the wrong foods, or not exercising enough. These messages were reinforced by people around me including medical professionals. My belief that the problem was me and the shame that went with it impacted on my ability to get help, and some of the beliefs I developed about myself during this time are things I still live with and work to overcome today.

I think one of the factors that contributes to the stigma surrounding endometriosis and my personal feelings of shame relates to the dominance of the medical model in the UK. When you present to a doctor with a problem, they will aim to find an explanation for that problem – a diagnosis. If no medical explanation can be found, then it can feel like no problem exists or that the problem is 'psychological'. Although naming someone's experience as having no medical explanation may be well intended, it is not one I experienced as helpful. Being told there was no medical explanation tended to be framed as no explanation existed for my symptoms, and I felt that they were therefore invalid and at times that they were not real. I was told that there was 'nothing wrong with me', that my periods were normal, and that I simply had a 'low threshold for pain'. The impact of being repeatedly told that your own experience is not valid or accurate is beyond words. You come to question your own reality and begin to conceal your experience from others fearing they will not understand. This reinforces shame and the belief that the problem is you.

CFT explains that humans are predisposed to experiencing shame, and we have brains that are evolved in a way that can get us caught up in tricky loops. If we can understand these loops and challenges, we may be able to take more control over the patterns that emerge in our thinking and behaviour. This model is one I have used to formulate my own experience and the experiences of my patients; and I hope you will be able to use to formulate your experience too.

Within this chapter, I hope to help you consider your distress differently and be able to disentangle some of the tricky loops you might find yourself stuck in. You are not the problem and nor are you solely responsible for the solution. The aim of this book is to help you bring together the difficulties you have with a range of coping strategies and actions that might be helpful. In other words, to formulate your distress.

Compassion-Focussed Therapy (CFT)

There are many models for formulating distress and mental health difficulties within psychological therapy. One of the first things you are taught about as a psychology student is the bio-psycho-social approach to care and to understand suffering, disease, and illness. This model has dominated industrialised societies since the mid-20th century (Engel, 1977) and was devised to challenge the disempowerment of patients that was one of the key criticisms of the biomedical model at the time. The biomedical model focussed on diagnosis of disease without consideration of the patient or their social world (Borell-Carrio et al., 2004). In contrast, the bio-psycho-social model was championed by sectors of the medical profession that wanted to bring more compassion to medical practice. The bio-psycho-social model suggests that a person's biology, psychology, and social context should be considered and integrated to fully assess, diagnose, and manage their difficulty and well-being. This approach forms part of the foundation of many psychological therapies. As a therapist building a formulation with a patient, you want to understand the context that they exist in and the factors that influence them. This can be their cultural background, their family, generational influences, religious beliefs, and many other elements of our lives.

When I was training as a clinical psychologist, we were introduced to several psychological models and therapies to enable us to develop formulations and treatment plans with our patients. Some therapies focus on a specific problem area, such as Cognitive Behavioural Therapy which has specific protocols for the treatment of trauma, anxiety, and depression alongside many others. However, my distress never fitted into a diagnosis or a category, so I didn't feel like the models I was learning as a trainee clinical psychologist quite fitted with what I was personally experiencing. This was until I was introduced to CFT during my clinical psychology training. I remember this teaching as a lightbulb moment, as the approach immediately felt like something that would be useful to me professionally, but it also resonated with my personal experience, and I began to learn more about this model so I could begin to apply the concepts to myself. In this book, I am taking the work of Paul Gilbert and colleagues from the Compassionate Mind Foundation and CFT resources and applying them to endometriosis based on my personal experience. These ideas and models are not my own, but the work of many others which I have been able to utilise personally, adapt for endometriosis, and share with you. The images presented in this chapter are provided by the compassionate mind foundation and I thank them for allowing me to share their work. You will find information on the work of the foundation and references to expand your knowledge of CFT at the end of this book.

CFT promotes an evolutionary and bio-psycho-social informed approach to compassion which forms the basis for CFT. It was developed by Paul Gilbert who, along with his colleagues, founded the Compassionate Mind Foundation in 2006. CFT focusses on developing compassion as a way of alleviating distress, particularly distress associated with high levels of self-criticism and shame.

Paul Gilbert has said that compassion is valuable because 'Compassion gives us the courage and wisdom to descend into our suffering' (The Compassionate Mind Foundation, 2023). I feel that living with endometriosis has fuelled my own descent into suffering many times. I lacked compassion to myself and did not always receive compassion from others, particularly medical professionals. Utilising the models and interventions from CFT has enabled me to connect with self-compassion, and this has changed how I relate to my own suffering. CFT has not stopped me from suffering or finding things difficult, and I personally believe that suffering is inevitable as a human being (a view that is also part of CFT). In addition, as endometriosis is an incurable disease, I anticipate needing to manage the suffering associated with it at other times in the future.

CFT provides an evidence-based model and treatment approach to understand why we find ourselves caught up in self-criticism and suffering (a formulation) which is presented in this chapter. It also utilises compassionate mind training to enable us to connect with compassion and to regulate our emotional systems differently. CFT did not, and could not, change the physical disease I had or the symptoms that went with it. However, it did help me to manage my suffering with care and connection rather than self-criticism and self-destruction.

The 'Tricky Brain'

One of the central ideas in CFT is the recognition that we all have tricky brains. Our brains have evolved in such a way that they leave us vulnerable to getting caught up in tricky loops that can cause and maintain our distress. The evolution of our brains has happened over millions of years, and we share parts of our brains with other animals such as reptiles and mammals. This part of our brain is called the old brain in CFT. There is also a part of our brain that has more recently evolved and has some uniquely human functions – this is called our new brain. These two parts of the brain have different functions – sometimes they work together and sometimes they work against each other in ways that can be unhelpful for us. Understanding the functions of our old and new brain and how the two parts work together can help us to notice tricky loops in ourselves.

Our old brain: Some of our brain structures exist to help us to navigate dangers in the world. We share some of these brain structures with reptiles and therefore this part of our brain is sometimes referred to as the 'reptilian brain'. Our old brain is motivated by survival – this includes food and reproduction as well as the fight, flight, freeze, and please/appease response that we will revisit later in this chapter. In our old brain, there is also a part that we share with other mammals. This is called the 'mammalian brain' which is motivated to engage in bonding with others, affection, play, and social communication.

Our new brain: As a species, we have developed a new part of our brain that is different to our ancestors and other animal species. This part of the brain is called the pre-frontal cortex, and it allows us to do all sorts of wonderful things. We can imagine things, consider the future, think about our thinking (sometimes called metacognition), and reflect on things in the past. These skills allow us to plan, navigate social relationships, form beliefs about our thoughts, and learn from things in our past.

Understanding Tricky Loops

Sometimes our old and new brains can interact well together and help us to reach our goals. However, at times they can also work against each other, causing us to get stuck in tricky loops. The diagram below adapted from Gilbert & Choden, 2022, shows how the old and new brain interact with one another.

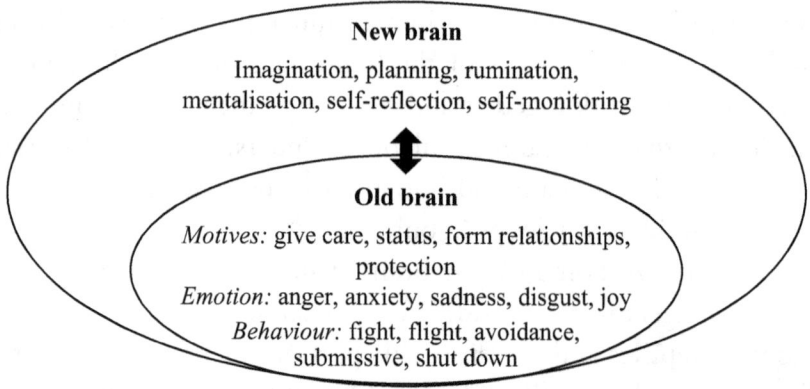

Old Brain/New Brain Interaction: from Gilbert, P., & Choden (2022) Mindful Compassion with permission from Little Brown. © P. Gilbert.

This is because our new brain can activate our old brain to think there is a threat, when we are in fact quite safe at that moment. I often have patients say 'I don't know why I am feeling this way' or 'I know this is just a thought, but I don't feel like it is.' This is because your brain is getting you caught up in a tricky loop. The thought produced by your new brain is activating a response in your old brain. Sometimes, the new brain might be focussing on our past or our future causing our old brain and body to respond in the present as if that thing we are imagining or remembering is actually happening in the here and now. This makes you feel in the present, exactly as you did in the past. This is a loop that can often be seen in relation to traumatic experiences we may have had in our lives. Here is an example of a tricky loop I experienced:

> I had a big presentation coming up that had taken weeks to prepare. I was due to stand in front of over 100 people to speak about my work. I checked my diary and saw I would be in the autumn phase of my cycle when the presentation was booked, only a couple of days before my period would be due. I felt my alarm system activate when I realised this – I felt sick and my heart started racing. That night, I couldn't sleep thinking about what I would do if I had to manage my period and the pain, whilst giving the presentation. I didn't want to cancel it, and my mind kept going over thoughts and images of standing in front of all those people, trying not to pass out from the pain or knowing that the blood was starting to come through my clothing. My body's alarm system kept sounding – my heart was faster, my thoughts kept racing, I felt tense all over like I needed to jump into action at any moment. As this anxiety continued, new thoughts came about why I couldn't cope with 'normal periods' like everyone else could, and I felt angry with myself for not coping better. After a while of feeling this way, another thought emerged that it didn't seem like everyone else was having to deal with what I was dealing with. This made me angry with other people for not understanding my experience but also more angry with myself. I was angry that I had not been able to tell anyone how I was feeling because of how they might react based on my experiences in the past.

New brain: What if my period comes the day of this important presentation
Old brain: Heart racing, nausea, body tension, anxiety
New brain: Maybe I will bleed through whilst I am presenting and not be able to get to the toilet
Old brain: Increasing anxiety
New brain: I am unable to cope with 'normal' life, I am weak and not good enough
Old brain: Anxiety, inferiority, and anger (self-directed)
New brain: No one understands how difficult it is to live like this, no one will understand
Old brain: Anger (outwards directed) and avoidance (of sharing with others)

Although we do share parts of our brain with other species, these tricky loops that leave us vulnerable to distress seem to be unique to us as humans. This is because we are able to maintain a state of threat even when the threat itself has gone. For example, an animal faced with a predator will run away and once they are safe, they will continue eating, drinking, or whatever it was they were doing before they had to run. For us as humans, even when we get to safety, we continue to go over the threat keeping it present by imagining what could have happened, what might happen next time, and so on. When we are in a tricky loop, it can be difficult to stop thinking in this way.

For me, living with endometriosis and persistent pain was characterised by a constant state of threat that existed regardless of whether I was on my period or not. Often there is a misconception that endometriosis is 'just a bad period' and outside of this, all is well. In my experience, even if your symptoms reduce outside of your period, psychologically you continue to feel under threat by the disease because your new brain thinks, imagines, remembers, and ruminates resulting in tricky loops in the present that maintain distress about the past and future.

The Three-Systems Model

CFT uses a three-systems model to understand how we manage our emotions and experiences. Thinking in these systems is something I have found helpful to make sense of my experience. It has helped me to know which system is being activated for me in different situations and later, how I might manage this. This is in part about trying to keep the systems in balance – like a three-legged stool. All the legs need to be able to hold weight, if one is not as well formed as the others, the stool will wobble and feel unsafe to use. It might even topple over sometimes. Each one of these systems has a function and a motivation. They are all trying to achieve something, and if I could understand what the system is trying to achieve, I found it easier to bring compassion to that system. Let's look at each one of these systems in turn.

A Psychological Understanding of Endometriosis

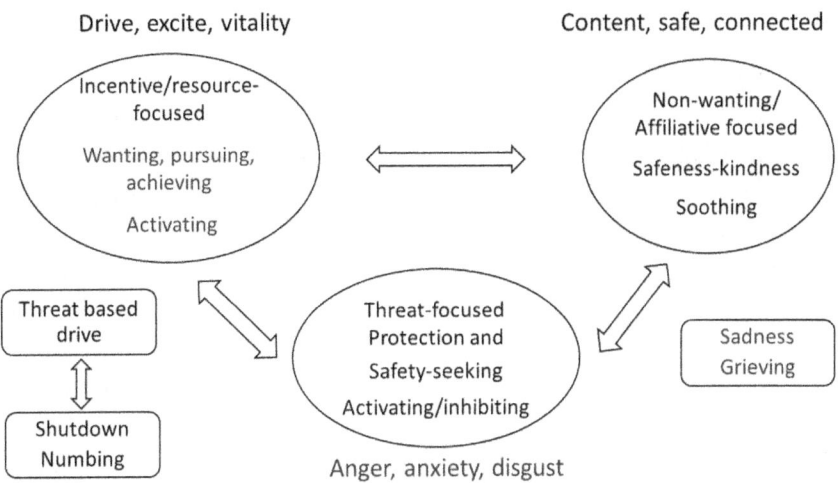

The Three Functions of Emotion: From Gilbert, P., & Simos, G. (2022). Compassion focused therapy: Clinical practice and applications, with permission from Routledge. Adapted from Gilbert, P. (2009) The Compassionate Mind, Little Brown. © P. Gilbert.

Threat and Self-Protection System

Many of us will have heard the term 'fight, flight, or freeze'. This is the basic premise of the threat system. This system's job is to identify threats quickly and then give us a signal (often a feeling such as fear or anxiety) to urge us to act against the threat – to protect ourselves and survive. We might be activated in this system to do something, for example, fight or flight. We might also be inhibited and freeze, which can mean we stop doing things or submit. It can also be activated if there are threats to the people we love or to the group we identify as belonging to. This is because we are a social species who survived due to our position in, and connection with, a group. Therefore, social threat is equivalent to other threats because being rejected from a group could result in us being left alone and dying. So, we have social threat responses that react in the same way as other life or death situations, and we carry these responses in the present from our evolved past. This system is motivated by survival and so takes a 'better safe than sorry' approach to the world.

I have worked with patients who label this system as negative, unpleasant, and unwanted because it is associated with feelings such as anger, anxiety, and disgust which can sometimes be difficult to experience and manage. However, we must remember that this system has evolved to protect us and that the brain is wired to pay more attention to threats than pleasurable things as the brain wants us to survive.

The Drive System

This system motivates us to seek out resources that we (and those important to us) need to thrive and survive. When balanced against the other two systems, the drive system guides us towards important life goals. When we achieve the goals we have set ourselves, our body releases the hormone dopamine which makes us feel happy and motivates us to continue to pursue our goals. However, sometimes our drive system can get out of balance. It might be underactive, and we then lack motivation and energy. Sometimes our drive system can become driven by our threat systems. This is called threat-based drive and can sometimes feel like the drive system is overactive, it can lead us to wanting more and more which is impossible to achieve and leads to feelings of frustration and disappointment. If we continue to be driven by our threat systems, then we may find ourselves falling into shutdown as we are tirelessly trying to achieve a goal which might be impossible to reach. Reaching a point of shutdown, or burnout, then activates our threat system.

Soothing and Contentment System

In his book *The Compassionate Mind*, Paul Gilbert says this system is difficult to describe. I would agree, but the way I describe it in therapy as the part of us that goes 'ahh'. Its job is to help us find a place of contentment – a place where we feel safe, just as we are, without striving or wanting. A place where we go 'ahh'.

This system relates to our relationship with ourselves and with others. It is linked to affection and kindness, which can be given to us by others. For example, when a parent comforts a child who is distressed, they are activating the soothing system for the child. This happens for us as adults too when we are comforted by other adults. We can also bring this comfort to ourselves through self-to-self compassion. When we move into our soothing systems, sometimes we may find feelings sadness and grief show up for us. These feelings can trigger threat, as they might relate to difficult or traumatic experiences which activate our threat systems. These feelings can also be difficult to manage at times and many of us are fearful of being overwhelmed by them. However, sadness and grief have a function and our soothing system can help us to navigate the threats associated with processing these painful emotions.

The Compassionate Mind

Through understanding our difficulties using CFT we work on developing a fourth circle that can sit in the middle of the three systems. We do this through compassionate mind training which allows us to learn new skills to develop our compassionate selves. This is a compassionate part of ourselves that can direct the flow of compassion across all our circles. It is a part of us that can hold a compassionate perspective and observe the three systems, working out a compassionate way to respond to what is happening. It is not about reducing or stopping our experience in any one of the three circles, but about bringing compassion to each system and its function. I found this particularly helpful in managing my experience because my threat system was often active. I was in pain every day, and this was debilitating at times – I became frustrated that my difficulties never went away completely and angry if others tried to soothe me by saying it would be OK or get better. Being able to bring compassion to my threat system and its function helped me to manage it differently.

Mapping Your Own Systems

One of the exercises I regularly use is mapping out my own emotional regulation systems. I find this helps me to recognise where I might be finding myself out of balance or what my body might be responding too at this point in time. First, it can be helpful to think about what you think your systems look like right now. You can use the space below to draw out the three circles. You might adjust the sizes in accordance with the dominance of that system in your life. When I started my journey, I think my systems looked like this:

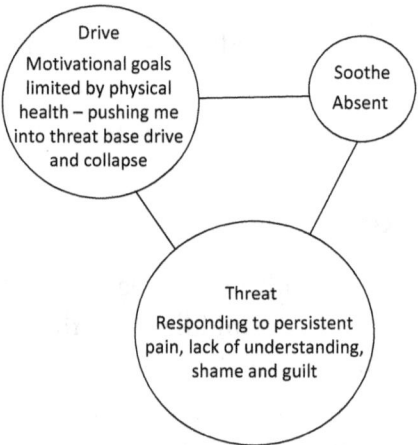

Space to draw your three systems

You might want to think about why your systems look like this right now. Whatever the reasons behind it, remember this is not your fault. Your systems have adapted to enable you to survive and to stay safe in the face of your struggles. The aim of this book is to help you create balance across all three systems and a compassionate centre that can direct compassion to all three parts.

I think my systems looked like the drawing here because I found it very difficult to step out of threat and drive to allow myself to soothe when I was younger. I was focussed on my goal of becoming a clinical psychologist and spent lots of time in threat based drive, working on gathering up experience and education that I believed would help me to reach this goal. However, sometimes it felt that the difficulties I had because of endometriosis blocked my healthy drive system and my ability to achieve my goals which pushed me back into threat or into a state of collapse. Pretty much everything about having endometriosis and suffering with it meant I was stuck in my threat system – most of the time. Even when I thought I was in drive, it was often a threat-based drive, focussing on the avoidance of threat rather than pleasure-seeking behaviour. Almost every achievement or life event I can think of that I wanted to be drive focussed, was tangled up in threat connected with the fears of what impact my illness might have on that goal or on that event. Rather than experiencing the buzz of feel-good hormone, like dopamine when I achieved something, I often just experienced frustration that I felt so physically unwell and emotionally drained afterwards, and I was exhausted by concealing just how difficult it all was.

For example, one of the symptoms associated with my endometriosis was interstitial cystitis and recurrent urinary tract infections. One of these progressed to a kidney infection that led to sepsis. I was extremely poorly at this time and was admitted to the high-dependency ward of our local hospital. I could not move and was on a bed that turned me to prevent bed sores. I had pneumonia and was on pressurised oxygen to support my lungs. My family were told that my prognosis was uncertain. As I lay in the high-dependency unit, I remember worrying that I wouldn't get my application in for clinical training that year (threat system activated) and asking my mum to bring me psychology textbooks to read in the hospital (threat-based drive). I was unable to lift my head most days – but the anxiety of being held back by my health, the shame of being lesser than others, and the knowledge that my health problems were ongoing activated my threat system to such an extent that I could not think rationally. My mum did not bring the books in, but I continued in this tricky loop of wanting to get back to work and moving towards the goal of applying for clinical training as quickly as possible. I was not compassionate to myself – I was critical of 'letting myself get ill' and 'failing to get better quickly enough'. I went back to work as quickly as I could, and my occupational health report documents concerns that my expectations of recovery were unrealistic. At the time, I believed I was in drive, focussed on achieving my goals, and saw this as a positive thing. However, I was really in threat and trying to mask this by pushing on which caused me more distress, both physically and emotionally. This was a pattern that repeated over many years in my life, and I am still working to avoid falling back into it now.

Living with chronic illness can mean spending a lot of time in threat, partly due to physical pain which also activates our threat system as our body tries to work out what is wrong. For me, it also meant framing things as positive, incentive-driven activities when they were sometimes motivated by an avoidance of threat or a fight response, because for a lot of the time I was angry. I was angry with myself because I kept being told there was nothing wrong with me and therefore I was angry I wasn't coping better – and I punished myself for it sometimes, withholding soothing because I didn't believe I needed it or deserved it– there wasn't anything wrong with me! Connecting with soothing can help us to regulate the physical threat response in our bodies (chapter 5), which can be helpful to keep our systems in balance. By avoiding soothing, I maintained threat in my body and in my mind – learning to activate my compassionate mind, and my soothing system was helpful in being able to connect with care and compassion from others and self-compassion.

If this is where you find yourself at present, withholding soothing and holding onto shame, I invite you to stop. For two minutes, just physically stop. Breathe and, if you can, ask yourself what system you are in and whether you need another system right now. You don't need to know how to get to that system; let's just start with knowing where you are and that there are other places to be. If you are stuck where I was, I want you to know you deserve more than that, and you are worth soothing. You can use the table below to think in more detail about each of the three systems and how they apply to you. This is adapted from the *Compassionate Mind Workbook (Irons & Beaumont, 2017)*.

	Threat System	Drive System	Soothing System
What parts of your experience activate this system? What brings it online?			
How do you know this system is activated? What happens?			
What do you want to do when this system is active?			
What emotions come up for you when this system is active?			

As you notice what your systems look like, you can begin to understand them better and make decisions about how to manage them. Through this book, we will continue to build on your understanding of these systems, their origins, and how they impact your difficulties now. We will also begin to work on developing your compassionate mind so you can connect with compassion in challenging times, enabling you to navigate that distress differently.

Summary

- Making sense of our experience can help us to consider the changes we might need to manage or even overcome our challenges. This is called a psychological formulation.
- CFT provides a model for us to make sense of our distress. It aims to help us use compassion to respond differently to our distress, hopefully reducing it.
- A compassionate approach may be helpful in addressing some of the tricky loops associated with shame and stigma in endometriosis.
- Tricky loops are patterns we can get caught up in because of how our brains have evolved (old brain, new brain). This is not our fault, but it can leave us vulnerable to distress.
- The three-systems model in CFT can help us to formulate our difficulties and think about how we might balance them. The skills we will learn in this book are aimed at helping us to develop a compassionate mind, which we can then use to connect with the flow of compassion in all three systems.
- When we understand our systems, we can then make decisions about how to approach them with compassion and find balance.

4   What Is Compassion and Why Is It Difficult?

What Is Compassion?

CFT defines compassion as:

> *A sensitivity to the suffering of self and others (and it's causes), with a commitment to relieve and prevent it. (Dale-Hewitt & Irons, 2015)*

Compassion is different to empathy or sympathy because it requires us to do something in response to our or other's distress. To be compassionate to someone (including ourselves), we need to connect with the suffering they are experiencing, and we need to want to do something to change it. Compassion is underpinned by hope that they will not feel this distress forever, regardless of how they are feeling in the present.

Engaging with distress, either our own or someone else's, can be a difficult thing to do. Sometimes other people's distress can be overwhelming, and we may want or need to distance ourselves from it. Sometimes, being compassionate to ourselves means putting in boundaries around how much we can be compassionate to other people and still be able to take care of ourselves. Striking this balance takes wisdom, courage, and a certain amount of skill. I have always been sensitive to the distress of other people. I remember crying over cartoon shows and getting involved with every charity fundraiser at school – my family labelled me a sensitive child as a result. When I declared my desire to become a clinical psychologist, my mum and grandmother both expressed concern that I would be too sensitive for a career with repeated exposure to distress. However, I think they missed a key element of being a clinical psychologist. You undergo years of training both to understand how to connect with distress and you develop professional skills and expertise to support people to take action to alleviate it. Learning to apply it to myself was a different journey, but one that has been essential personally and professionally. In this chapter, we will think about the qualities of compassion, the flows of compassion, and I will introduce you to some of the skills we are going to learn later in the book.

Qualities of Compassion

It might sound easy to begin to use compassion towards ourselves and others. However, it can be very challenging! We may have already defined compassion (Dale-Hewitt & Irons, 2015), but what does that look like in ourselves and our lives? What makes someone compassionate, and how can we embody compassion ourselves?

You can probably think of a person, real or fictional, that you think is compassionate. Chances are that this person has certain qualities about them that means you have picked them out over and above everyone else you could have thought of.

In CFT, we are looking to bring together the qualities that make up compassion alongside the skills needed to bring compassion to ourselves and to others. It can be helpful to understand more about the qualities of compassion, so we can begin to work on these in ourselves.

Paul Gilbert illustrates the qualities of compassion using a compassion circle. This incorporates both qualities and skills which will form the foundation of the later chapters of this book where we will think about how we bring together the qualities of compassion and specific skills to manage the symptoms of endometriosis.

The compassion circle shows an inner ring referring to the qualities of compassion and an outer ring referring to skills. In this chapter, I am going to spend some time thinking about the qualities of compassion and introduce some of the skills that we will be revisiting in later chapters.

What Is Compassion and Why Is It Difficult?

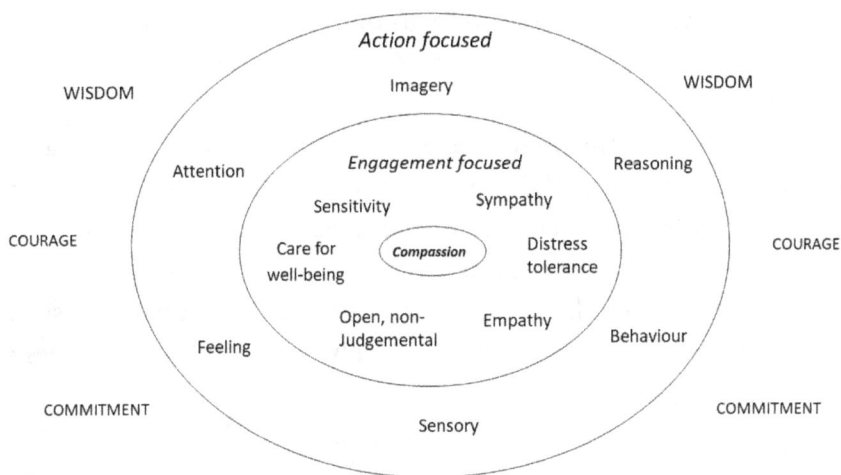

Domains for the Therapeutic Process. From Gilbert, P., & Simos, G. (2022). Compassion focused therapy: Clinical practice and applications, with permission from Routledge. Adapted from Gilbert, P. (2009) The Compassionate Mind, Little Brown. © P. Gilbert.

CFT suggests there are six core qualities that make up compassion. These six qualities, shown in the inner circle of the image, are engagement focused attributes of compassion. It argues that although there may be many other qualities to compassion, these six help us to engage with distress (the first part of compassion).

Sensitivity: Being able to tune into distress either our own or someone else's. Rather than blocking out or moving away from our difficulties, we are being open to noticing our emotions, thoughts, feelings, and behaviours.

Sympathy: In CFT, sympathy means being emotionally moved by our own, or other people's, distress. For example, you might feel sympathy for someone on a TV show who is going through emotional pain. Sympathy is important because it can be the precursor to taking action to alleviate suffering. Being sympathetic to your own pain is a step towards self-compassion. For me, I found it very difficult to be sympathetic to my own suffering.

Care for well-being: Trying to focus on a part of us that cares about this, that is motivated to find ways of dealing with our own or others' distress in helpful ways.

Non-judgement: The ability to accept, without judgement, that we all have tricky brains and can get caught up in loops that are unhelpful. Acting without judgement does not mean being passive and excusing the behaviour of yourself or others. However, it does mean being able to move out of threat and away from our own self-criticism to try to think more clearly about what might be helpful for ourselves or others in any given situation.

Empathy: Empathy is 'feeling with people' (Brene Brown, RSA Short, 2013) – being able to imagine the experiences of others and consider what is behind them behaving in a certain way or expressing a certain feeling. Feeling with people is more difficult than feeling sympathy for someone, as feeling with people requires you to consider and connect with a perspective that might be different to your own. This can be challenging and sometimes painful.

Distress Tolerance: Being more attuned to your own distress can be difficult. It is therefore important to learn how that distress and difficult feelings will pass and how to tolerate our distress whilst it is present.

You may want to think about whether any of these qualities are already present for you and which might be more difficult or challenging. I found it very difficult to approach myself without judgement at the peak of the illness, and I found it impossible to connect with my own distress at times, for fear I would be overwhelmed by it. This was most noticeable in relation to managing persistent and severe pain. In chapter 7, we will think more about the qualities of compassion and how we can build these into our compassionate selves.

Part of developing distress tolerance in myself came from beginning to learn skills to help me manage that distress, which lessened the fear that I would not be able to cope with it as I felt more in control when I had strategies in place to manage it. In each of the forthcoming chapters, I am going to outline some of the central difficulties I had with endometriosis, and I will then share some of the skills I found helpful in relation to those difficulties. I feel that it would be helpful to give an overview of those skills here, so you can begin to familiarise yourself with some of the central ideas.

The Flows of Compassion

There are three flows of compassion: from others to self, from self to others, and from self to self. Some flows of compassion might be easier for you than others. I find it much easier to give compassion (self-to-other compassion) than to receive it (other-to-self compassion), especially from myself (self-to-self compassion). I have also learnt that when I open myself up to receiving compassion from other people, I feel stronger and less alone.

Let's start with thinking about the flow of self to others. This can be a helpful starting point to explore connecting with compassion as we can then consider whether we give this same compassion that we show to others towards ourselves. The example below was a frequent dilemma I faced when living with endometriosis – completing everyday tasks during a period. As you read the example, imagine this person (me in this case) is your friend or loved one and think how you might respond to them in a compassionate way. I have used my own name and experience for the example.

> *Kirsty's period had been particularly heavy this month – she had been bleeding heavily for ten days and felt exhausted. The cramps had meant she had not been able to sleep, and this was making her feel even worse. It was Friday night and Kirsty had planned to do her food shopping and washing ready for the weekend. Kirsty gives you a call before she is going out that evening to talk to you about her week and her plans. She is unsure whether to go shopping tonight but is putting pressure on herself to get things done.*
>
> *How might you respond to her?*

_____
_____
_____
_____

Hopefully, you have responded to Kirsty with kindness and wisdom, which are some of the qualities of compassion we have identified in this chapter. Perhaps you have helped her come up with alternative solutions to her dilemma, such as online shopping or asking someone for help. Being compassionate towards another person (self to other) is likely to make that person feel cared for, listened to, and supported at this difficult time. This may help to activate their soothing system so they can manage their own distress differently.

Many of us find it easier to show compassion to others (self to others) than to receive compassion from others (other to self). We are hardwired to want and need compassion from others to navigate our struggles in life. Unfortunately, common responses to people living with endometriosis are often significantly lacking in compassion, perhaps due to the lack of understanding of the disease. Research from the Alliance for Endometriosis showed that 90% of people with endometriosis report being dismissed, disbelieved, or ignored by other people. Even if people can look towards your suffering, they may lack the knowledge or resources to be able to help you manage it, and this might mean they turn away. I think this can happen sometimes in relationships with partners, friends, and family and with ourselves. Sometimes not knowing what to do, or understanding what is happening, means it can be easier to ignore it rather than embrace the suffering without a solution.

Receiving compassion from others can be a difficult and overwhelming experience, and we will discuss some of the challenges in more detail in the barriers section of this chapter. For me, I personally felt I did not deserve compassion from others because I was failing to cope with something that everyone else could deal with easily. I remember occasions when people would say 'you need to give yourself some time, rest and recover'. They would offer to help me to allow me the space to slow down. I found it difficult to accept this, saying I was fine or giving excuses as to why I couldn't stop. Often these related to other people, for example, not taking time off work because I didn't want to let anyone down or for anyone to have to cover for me. I felt many threats competing with one another, and it was difficult to know what to prioritise. This continues to be a pattern I find hard to overcome. However, if we can be open to the kindness and support of others, it can have significant effects on our brains and bodies, which can help us to regulate our three systems.

In addition to connecting with the flow of others to self to manage our distress we can also connect with self-compassion (self to self), as this is essential for our well-being. Think back to the example from earlier – when you thought about how you would respond to Kirsty, is this also how you would respond to yourself in a similar situation, or do you notice yourself responding to yourself in a different way?

Self-compassion refers to the ability to direct compassion towards ourselves, something which I found difficult (and sometimes impossible) when living with endometriosis. Self-to-self compassion felt to me like the hardest skill to master. Like many people, I sometimes felt being compassionate to myself would be letting the illness win because I was stuck in threat-based drive so taking time to stop and rest, got in the way of achieving my goals and that felt like failure. I think that is because to be compassionate to myself required an acceptance that I was finding things difficult, something I was loathed to admit, even to myself as my drive system which wanted to be independent and strong was being contaminated by threat. I convinced myself that I was already being quite compassionate to myself for many years of my illness, but when I learnt more about CFT I realised this wasn't the case. More times than not, I was avoiding being compassionate to myself and waiting until my freeze response kicked in to take any time for myself at all. When I reached this point, I was not able to be compassionate to myself or others as I had reached total burn out, a collapse response. There was no skill in this approach – no active attempts to alleviate my suffering. I just pushed myself until suffering took over.

Barriers to Compassion

Whenever I speak, read, or learn about compassion and compassionate behaviour, I often feel that it sounds like it is an easy thing to do. Be compassionate to yourself and other people – problem solved! I have struggled with the conflict between knowing about these ideas and their value professionally, but personally struggling to apply them. I am not alone in this – many people find there are barriers to compassion.

In CFT, these barriers are called fears, blocks, and resistances. These can be grouped together as FBRs because they are all threat responses to a certain type of compassion (other to self, self to others, or self to self). In this book, we will look at FBR's as a group because in my own experience, I found they were often mixed up with one another. FBRs are something we might all experience at different times and for different reasons. These may develop from, or be rooted in, our past life experiences. It is not our fault that these FBRs have developed for us, but it is our responsibility to work through them. FBRs disrupt the three flows of compassion (self to self, self to others, others to self), and it is important to understand them so we can prevent them from continuing to get in the way of our connection with compassion and reduction in our distress. As we work through FBRs, it is important to remember what we discussed in chapter 3 – we all get caught up in tricky loops. It is not your fault that you may be fearful of compassion. Some of us share similar fears because of living with endometriosis and the distress it may have bought into our lives.

We will think about FBRs to each flow of compassion here. As you read through these, try thinking about the possible FBRs that might be relevant to you.

Fear of giving compassion to others can be associated with worries that we may be taken advantage of, or it might have a negative impact on our well being or resources to connect with the distress of another person. I would not identify myself as someone who usually experiences fear relating to giving compassion to others. However, when writing this book, I have thought in more depth about these themes in my endometriosis journey and noticed that this fear was present for me. I often wondered whether I would find it helpful to connect with other people with the condition, but I didn't utilise online support groups for years, and I never attended any face-to-face support groups. I feel this was because I felt unable to connect with others who were also suffering when I was stuck in threat myself. Although I think not joining a support group was right for me at that time, I am mindful that I did feel isolated for much of my illness, and this might have been exacerbated by not wanting to be in a face-to-face situation with other people also experiencing similar struggles. I also struggled with opening myself up to the compassion of others as a person who was suffering. Although I utilised online support, I wouldn't post myself, but would search for people having a similar experience to me and read those comments. My fear was that if I posted something myself people might not show compassion to me and that prevented me from opening up.

Fear of receiving compassion from others can be rooted in mistrust. This might be from our past experiences, for example, being repeatedly hurt or abandoned by others or feeling that others would not meet our needs in a compassionate way. During my school years I experienced bullying and this impacted my ability to trust others during my teenage years and into my early adulthood. I had difficulties trusting medical professionals after repeated experiences of feeling let down and misunderstood at times I was vulnerable. This fear can mean we put up a barrier to other people, to protect ourselves from being let down. Although this makes sense, it can prevent us from getting the help and support we need.

My mistrust of healthcare professionals meant that when they did offer me compassion, my threat system would become active. My overwhelming experience of contact with healthcare professionals was one where I was not believed, where I was repeatedly dismissed, and where I was left feeling that my experiences were in my head or a reflection of my own inability to cope with a normal period. This created an FBR where I would avoid seeing healthcare professionals at times because of fear of how I would be treated. When I met compassionate healthcare staff (and there were many), I was suspicious of them. The consultant who did my hysterectomy surgery was one of the most compassionate people I met in my journey. He made me feel that my experience was valid, and I trusted him to complete my surgery. His support allowed me to confront some of the the FBRs that were still getting in the way of my compassion to self – that I did not believe my experience was real. Being believed by this consultant and his efforts to do everything he could to help me, helped me to believe that perhaps I was deserving of help and gave me some permission to help myself in ways I had not considered previously.

I asked him to go through the images of my surgery with me after the operation. This was because after years of suffering and being told there was nothing wrong, I needed to see for myself what was happening inside me. I knew he believed me, and he would talk me through the surgery, but this did not feel enough. I needed to see the images for myself and understand them. When he talked me through the images, I was overwhelmed with emotion. Although I was horrified at the extent of my endometriosis and the extent of the surgery, I was also thankful that there was proof that I had endometriosis – finally an explanation for my decades of suffering. I kept those images because this was the first time I had really been able to say to myself 'it's understandable you are struggling, you are not weak and you deserve kindness' – a connection with self-to-self compassion.

Fear of giving compassion to self can occur for a wide range of reasons rooted in our previous experiences. We may have learnt that we don't deserve to receive compassion, or that being compassionate to ourselves makes us weak. We might find it difficult to identify what our own needs are and therefore not know how to meet them. Common themes here might be 'I will be giving in/letting myself off the hook', or 'I am weak', or 'if I am compassionate to myself, I won't achieve anything.' All of these were present for me. I was terrified that if I was compassionate to myself, I would be unable to do anything. This was partly because I saw compassion as stopping me from achieving things, rather than connecting me with something helpful. I feared I would lose my career, my friendships, my relationships, and my hobbies. This was exacerbated by my awareness that my illness was chronic and incurable. As an example, I found it difficult to rest because I knew I wasn't going to recover through rest. I was going to continue to be ill and in pain, so I continued to ignore my own needs and keep going as an avoidance of connecting with the distress of being in pain and needing to rest because of this. Not only did this get in the way of compassion for self, but it was also another factor that impacted my ability to receive compassion from others as I concealed much of what I was going through at that time from other people as well as denying it to myself.

Understanding the Origins of Our Fears and Their Unintended Consequences

As discussed in chapter 3, clinical psychologists focus on formulation as a way of deepening our understanding of our experiences and the challenges we face. In this chapter, you may have begun to identify some of the FBRs that might get in the way of the three flows of compassion for you. As we discussed earlier, some FBRs can be rooted in our experiences which have occurred throughout our lives. These experiences activate our threat system and our fears, so we develop ways of coping with this. These are called protective or safety strategies. These strategies have been developed by our brains to try to reduce threat and to keep us safe. However, our brain is tricky, and it doesn't always find strategies that are effective in the long term. This can result in unintended consequences that might be unhelpful.

In CFT, there is a tool called a four-part formulation to help us think about the links between our past experiences, our fears, our safety strategies, and their unintended consequences in more detail. In chapter 3, we looked at our three systems and how these relate to one another. This exercise helps us to focus in on our fears and safety strategies so we can understand why we get caught up in behaviours that might have unintended consequences which are unhelpful to us in the longer term. I have presented my version of this below.

COPING WITH ENDOMETRIOSIS

Key Past Experiences	Key Fears/Threats	Protective/Safety Strategies	Unintended Consequences
Repeated contact with healthcare providers from the age of 12 who dismissed my experience Not being educated about periods in any detail and therefore not understanding that some periods were not normal	I will not be listened to Other people would not help me/respond to me with compassion	Avoid seeing healthcare professionals where possible Minimise my experience with other people Avoid talking about my experience with others	Symptoms worsened without correct treatment Other people did not understand what I was experiencing, so I felt more isolated, alone, and misunderstood Anger and irritability with others for not understanding/often being intolerant of others
Learning that periods were normal and something that I should be able to manage Seeing other people seemingly cope well with periods	If I do not do what is expected of me, or is the same as other people, this will be the evidence of my weakness. Other people will think I am exaggerating/lying and be angry with me	Hide my experience from others Push myself to continue as normal despite pain or distress Criticise myself for my feelings and difficulties	Increased pain, exhaustion, and distress Lack of support, increased isolation Stuck in self-criticism, increasing my shame

There is a blank version of this below which you can complete to think about your own patterns. In the next part of this chapter, we will then think about how you might begin to develop some of the qualities and skills associated with compassion so you can begin to change these patterns.

Key Historical Influences	Key Fears/ Threats	Protective/Safety Strategies	Unintended Consequences

Introduction to Skills

CFT refers to the development of skills as compassionate mind training – this is because we are trying to train our brains to behave in a more compassionate way. This is not an easy task and takes time to achieve. As we begin to learn these new skills, we will think about how to implement them into daily life. With any new skill, it is helpful to repeat it, and I find this is more achievable if it is done in small bursts as often as possible. It is important that you do what works for you. You will have strengths and things that you enjoy, so we want to try to build on these things as you learn something new rather than trying something that doesn't feel right for you. Throughout this book, I am going to share with you the ideas from CFT to try. Some might feel right for you, and some might not. You are welcome to pick and choose as we go through what you want to experiment with – start with the things you feel you can use. You might come back to skills that might be more challenging later. That's OK – go with what works!

These are some of the key things we are going to be thinking about in later chapters.

Compassionate attention: Our tricky loops mean we can all get caught up at times focussing on things that keep us stuck in threat, often without us even noticing. It is only recently that I have begun to appreciate how often I was caught up by my own loops and stuck in my threat system. Compassionate attention is learning to direct our attention in a particular way with a compassionate focus. These skills are also part of mindfulness.

Compassionate imagery: We have talked about how imagery can be very powerful in activating different systems for us. In the same way our threat system might be triggered by a memory of something that was difficult for us, we can also use imagery to create compassion-specific images. This might be memories we are bringing to mind, or it might be things we have imagined or created to use at times of distress.

Compassionate reasoning: This is the alternative to spending lots of time caught up in tricky loops. It's a way of training our minds to think differently about ourselves, other people and the situations we find ourselves in. This can be done by asking ourselves questions to guide our thinking in different ways. Often these are the kinds of questions I would ask my patients as a clinical psychologist to try to guide their thinking, so in a way, this is your own inner therapist trying to support you to move your thinking. This might include looking at the alternative perspective, weighing up the evidence or opening up your thinking.

Compassionate behaviour: Compassionate behaviour is using our wise minds to work out what actions are going to be helpful to alleviate our own, or someone else's distress or suffering. This includes setting boundaries for ourselves and others and understanding that sometimes what is compassionate in the short term may not be in the long term. You make a commitment to act in a compassionate way, even if this is not how you feel in that moment. This can help with activating your drive system.

Compassionate feelings: This is focussing on building up positive emotions and tolerating distress. This can include love, kindness, warmth, patience, and wisdom.

As you will see, there are lots of ways we can develop our compassionate minds. In this book, we are going to think about how these different skills may be helpful to manage the psychological impact of living with endometriosis. This is something that you will build up as you work through this book and you practice the things you learn from it. I encourage you to pace yourself. You might find that you spend more time working on the skills from some chapters than others. Remember to take the time you need to work on these skills – it is not easy, and you may be trying to learn them whilst you are in threat and suffering yourself. Take your time – you will get there.

Summary

- Compassion is defined as being sensitive to the distress of ourselves and others, with a commitment to relieve and prevent that distress.
- Compassion flows in three directions: from others to self, self to others, and self to self. It can be helpful to think about whether the compassion we direct to others is the same or different as the compassion we direct towards ourselves.
- There are many barriers to compassion, and it is helpful to understand the barriers that might get in the way of you connecting with compassion so you can work to overcome these barriers.
- Barriers to compassion are sometimes referred to as fears, blocks, and resistances (FBRs).
- Some FBRs may be connected to our past experiences, and we can use a four-part formulation to explore the connections between our past experiences and our present difficulties. This

can also help us understand why we behave in the way we do and the unintended consequences of this behaviour.
- There are several qualities of compassion, and CFT aims to bring together the qualities of compassion with skills so we can connect with our compassionate minds and the three flows of compassion.
- This book contains skills to connect us with compassion as we navigate the journey of coping with endometriosis.

5   Understanding Threat

The Body's Response to Threat

When we looked at threat in chapter 3, we noted that our threat system is activated when it identifies something that could pose a threat to us or to those around us. We cannot turn it off or make it go away completely because it is there for a reason.

Remember that the threat system is designed to keep us safe in the face of possible or confirmed danger. It is trying to be helpful by letting us know that a threat might be present, and this might need us to respond so we can stay safe. We can make sense of this when we think about how we have evolved as a species, starting with our prehistoric ancestors. Imagine you are a prehistoric human, you come out of your lovely cave where you are confronted by a huge animal. This animal is bigger than you, it is hungry, and it is vicious. Your threat system needs to be activated in response to this animal, so that you can take action to keep yourself (and others) safe.

This is an example of an external trigger. Something that happens external to us that our brains view as a threat to our safety. So, our brain alerts us, saying 'watch out, there's danger' and sending signals to our body to cause a response as quickly as possible to keep us safe (by running away, for example). This is an unconscious process – it happens so quickly we are barely even aware of it, and it can take our conscious mind a few seconds to make sense of what is happening.

I like to think about the body's response to threat like an alarm system. We can think about a smoke alarm as an example. Like a smoke alarm, our body's alarm system can be activated by anything that might be a threat. It works on the rule that it is 'better safe than sorry'. However, like a smoke alarm, this can lead to lots of false alarms – where our body is responding to things it thinks are a threat but turn out not to be (like burnt toast). And, like a smoke alarm, if our body's alarm goes off, we need to respond to it. This might be just confirming that this is a false alarm, and no further action is needed, or it might be more significant action to keep ourselves safe. Sometimes this will be easy, and we can quickly bring down and silence the alarm, other times it can be more difficult. In this chapter, we will consider both how the alarm system goes off in our body and how we can begin to respond to it in a way that helps us to manage it.

When our senses detect a possible threat, they send a signal to a part of our brain called the amygdala which assesses the information. If the amygdala thinks this information that it has been given by our senses might be a threat, it sends a signal to another part of the brain called the hypothalamus which sends a signal to our nervous system.

If our threat response is like an alarm, then our nervous system is like a volume control. There is a sympathetic nervous system, which turns up the alarm – this allows us to know that we must act now, and it also gives us resources to be able to act. There is also a parasympathetic nervous system which turns the alarm down and off – this system allows us to recover from the alarm and our response to it.

When our alarm system is activated, and the volume is going up, adrenaline is released by our body. This results in physical changes in the body, which are designed to help us in the short term. Here's an example of what that might feel like.

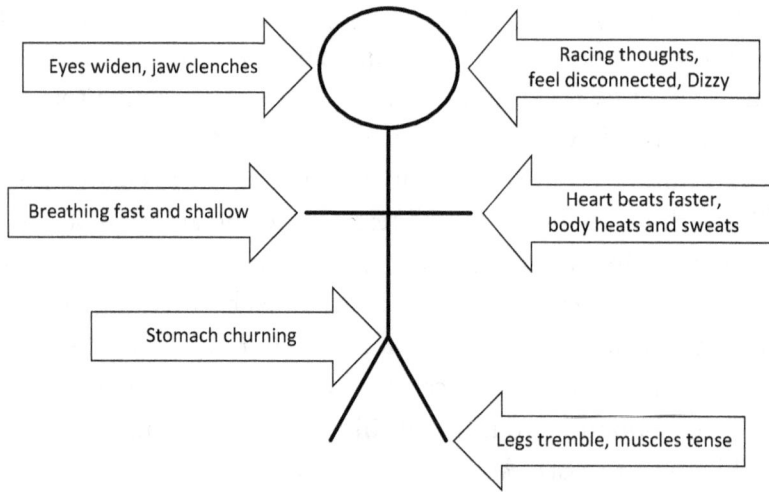

Understanding Threat

Now take a moment to think of how this might feel for you. It can be helpful to pick a recent situation in which you felt stressed – this may or may not be related to your endometriosis. Try adding onto the picture below the physical experiences you noticed in your body at this time. I have put an example of how I notice threat showing up in my body in the table on the left, and you can add yours on the right or on the stick person. You may experience some of the same things that I do, but you might not. That is OK as this experience is different for everyone. There can also be a difference between what we feel in a moment of acute stress and what it feels like being under chronic stress long term. You may want to try to think about this as you complete the exercise.

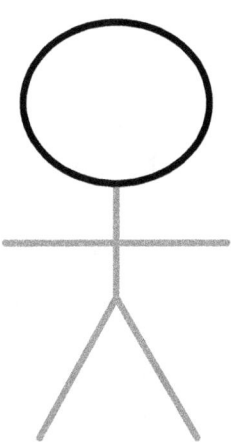

MINE	YOURS
Headache or migraine	
Blurry vision/feeling eye strain	
Heart rate increase – palpitations	
Feeling cold – sensation of heart dropping	
Dry mouth – swallowing a lot	
Tummy discomfort – needing to go to the toilet more than usual	

Once we identify how threat shows up in our body, this can help us to make sense of it and begin to address it. This can be particularly challenging in endometriosis as you may be experiencing many physical symptoms at the same time, some might be acute (a sudden, loud alarm), and some might be chronic (a constant alarm you try to ignore). Persistent pain might make you feel disconnected from your body at times as you try to tune out to the alarm as you feel unable to control it. The problem here is that you might be tuning out to other signals too. What we need to be able to do is pull apart possible symptoms of the condition from a threat response, as this enables us to choose how to respond to what is happening.

Triggering the Threat Response

Now that you understand what happens in your body when your threat response is activated, you need to identify the triggers behind this response. The word 'triggered' is often used on social media to explain the experience we are discussing here. When we say we are triggered, we mean we have experienced a strong physical and/or emotional response to something. The something that has triggered us can be external or internal. Both internal and external triggers can provoke the same threat response in our bodies (think back to tricky loops where we talked about new brain triggering the old brain response).

Earlier in this chapter, we looked at examples of an external trigger. An external trigger is something that comes from the world around us, for example, a person, a place, a situation, a sound, or a smell. We are all triggered by external threats that threaten our survival – like that hungry animal that wants to eat us. However, other external threats can be specific to our experience and develop over time or in response to things that have happened to us. This can explain why some of us find certain situations manageable and some of us find them terrifying, for example, hospitals.

As well as external triggers that make us feel afraid, there can be internal triggers that activate our threat response. Internal triggers come from inside us. This might be a memory, a thought, a feeling, or a physical sensation. Like external triggers, we notice these experiences, and our brain responds to let us know that there could be a threat. A common example of this for me would have been cramping pains – if I experienced a cramping pain, my threat response would be activated as I became anxious about what was happening. It might be that I hadn't started my period and I would worry about it starting particularly if I was in an environment that made the possibility of bleeding feel more unsafe, for example, a public place with limited access to a toilet. In this situation, there would be an overlap between internal and external triggers which made the experience more stressful and threatening. This is also an example of the old brain, new brain tricky loops we discussed in chapter 3. The new brain imagines that the cramp indicates bleeding or the start of a flare up, which makes our old brain and our body respond as if it is happening even though it might not be.

There are many experiences I can think of from living with endometriosis where there was an overlap between both internal and external triggers. Many of those relate to feelings of embarrassment and shame, for example, fear that people would see blood on my clothes, or I would have a flare up in public and faint. We are going to think more about the role of shame in chapter 6, but let's make the link between threat and shame here.

Triggers are not always life or death situations; they can also be things that cause us to feel embarrassed or ashamed. This is because we humans have evolved to belong to a group. We place a lot of value on social relationships and belonging. In part, this is because our chances of survival are increased if we belong to a group. We can share resources and take care of one another as we would in a tribe. We still use the word and concept of belonging to a tribe in modern-day life as we surround ourselves with people who share the same values as us. It is difficult for us to survive in isolation, both physically and mentally. It makes sense then that we would be threatened by things that might mean we will be rejected by others or left out of a social group. This is a very old threat which is wired into our modern brains and still gets activated in the here and now, as social rejection in the past could have eventually led to our death because our ancestors needed a group to survive. I experienced the threat of people knowing about my experience and judging me for it as one of the most difficult things about living with endometriosis.

Living with endometriosis meant I developed a sensitivity to internal and external triggers that might not have been present for me without this experience. My experience of problem periods started when I was young and contributed to how I understood the world, myself, and other people. We all develop ways of coping with our experiences (see your four-part formulation from earlier). These responses make us feel safe in that moment but can have unintended consequences. We are going to think later in this chapter about some of our built-in responses to threat and how they can influence our behaviour.

Part of being able to use the techniques we are learning together in this book is knowing the possible internal and external experiences that might trigger our threat response. This can bring a degree of predictability to our experience, and we can then prepare ourselves and choose the skills that are going to help us manage that trigger. The key to this technique is becoming better at telling the difference between when our alarm system is responding to burnt toast and when it is responding to a fire.

Threat Responses – Strategies to Keep Us Safe in Response to Threat

When the body's alarm system is triggered, it is trying to get us to respond. Like a smoke alarm, if we ignore it, it will continue to alert us to the possible danger. It may even continue to get louder over time until we respond to it or are overwhelmed by it completely.

The body's responses to threat can be grouped into four categories. Most people can name three of them – the fight, flight, and freeze responses. There is also a please or appease response, which is where we might do or go along with what someone else thinks or wants to reduce danger. Like the physical symptoms we experience when faced with a trigger, our responses to triggers are also hard-wired. They are survival strategies that we will all implement at various times in our lives to keep ourselves safe. However, these strategies are designed to help us at times of acute stress (threat) and are not designed for long term use. Long term exposure to stress can impact our physical and mental health in negative ways. If living with endometriosis is part of the source of this stress, then it may not be possible to eliminate the stress completely, but we may be able to reduce its impact in other ways.

When the threat system is activated, we will respond to it in a way that makes us feel safer in that moment. If you think back to the four-part formulation from chapter four, you may have already identified some of the safety strategies you have put in place to manage your threat response. These strategies might fall into the categories outlined by 'fight, flight, freeze, please/appease', or they might be different. These responses are designed to be helpful and allow us to react quickly so we can stay safe. However, sometimes they can have unintended consequences (as outlined in chapter 4).

Let's think about each response in turn and how this might show up in endometriosis.

Flight Response: This helps us to escape from a threatening situation by preparing our body for physical activity (running, for example). Our heart rate and breathing get faster, our muscles get tenser, and our thinking and attention are sharpened so we can focus on ways to escape. I often felt the flight response at times of high anxiety, when I wanted to run away from the situation I was faced with. Most often this was hospital admissions or surgeries as I did not want to be in the hospital environment where I felt powerless and out of control. I had to learn to manage my flight response (and not run away!) so I could have the treatment I needed. In its more subtle form, flight might look like keeping busy to avoid danger (a form of running away by avoidance).

Fight Response: The fight response may be a risky strategy, as it comes with the possibility we could lose, resulting in injury to us. However, if we win our chances of survival are increased. Like the flight response, our body prepares for physical activity in the same way and our attention focuses on danger. Living with endometriosis never required me to enter physical fights with another person. However, there were situations where I did become angry with others and I did feel like I was fighting to get myself heard and to access the care I needed. Fight also shows up for me in other ways such as being irritable and intolerant of others and finding it difficult to concentrate on a task or on information being given to me.

Freeze Response: The freeze response aims to make us less noticeable to the threat and may be our best chance of survival. In its early stages, the freeze response is designed to buy us some time – initially our thinking is quicker, and attention is more focussed. However, if prolonged, the freeze response can also lead to 'out of body' experiences, such as numbness to emotion and feeling disconnected from reality. This is sometimes called dissociation. For a long time, my primary response to threat was to freeze. I would shut down and wait for the threat (my period, for example) to go away. In the early stages of my endometriosis, this was more successful as the threat was time-limited but as the condition progressed and my symptoms became chronic, this strategy quickly became ineffective. I still find myself wanting to freeze and hide away at times of significant stress.

Please/Appease Response: If the threat is another person, giving them what they want (pleasing them) can reduce the danger. The unintended consequence here is that we might later regret our decision to please or we may have pleased someone at the cost of our own wellbeing. This is because in this moment, our mind is focussing on the option that might reduce the immediate threat and you might not 'see' the alternative options until after the threat has passed. During a please/appease response, we might try to make ourselves seem smaller to show we are appeasing the other person. This might be physically changing our posture (head down, shoulders rounded) or changing our voice (speaking quietly or not at all). Sometimes I noticed myself using this strategy as a pre-cursor or alternative to the fight response in my interactions with medical professionals. There were many appointments where I went in with the intention of advocating for myself, but instead found myself putting my head down and nodding along with what was being said by the doctor, even though I did not agree with it. I felt too afraid to say anything different and would leave the appointment feeling upset and frustrated. It was also a strategy I used to manage the impact of my disease on others around me – I would often go along with things that were very difficult because I didn't want others to judge me or reject me. Hiding my experience to please others remains a safety strategy that I work hard to change.

Sometimes the strategy we use is connected to the level of threat we are experiencing, but sometimes our response can be disproportionate to the trigger. I think it is helpful to understand that threat has a limit – a peak. That peak can be a terrifying place to be, but it can help to hold in mind that what goes up, must come down. If or when you do find yourself in the peak of anxiety, it may be that you cannot implement skills at this point and that the best you can do is to survive that experience as you wait for your anxiety to come down, and you can begin to regulate yourself again.

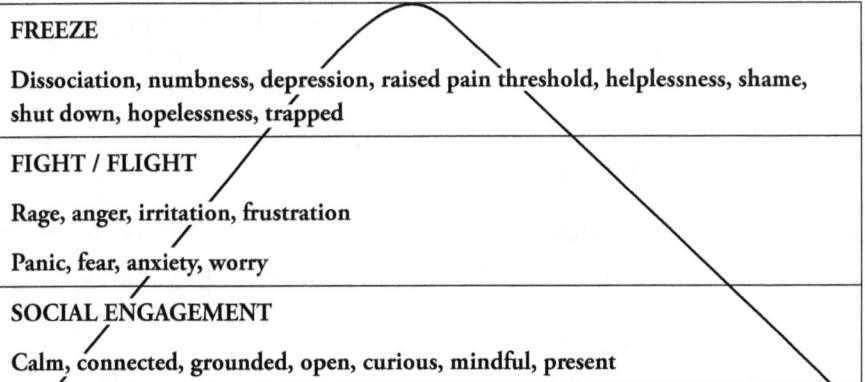

In this diagram, we can see how the things we have discussed so far in this chapter link together. When we are feeling safe, we are at the bottom of the curve. We can feel calm, content, and grounded. It is easy for us to engage with other people and the world around us.

If our threat response is activated, we might start to move up the curve as our alarm system starts getting louder. This can take different amounts of time and we may not always get to the top of the curve. When our alarm system is activated, we move into a state of hyperarousal. This is where we can hear our alarm loud and clear, it may even begin to get louder triggering our fight, flight, or please response. If it is our fight response we feel here, our emotions might be anger, irritation, or rage. If it is our flight response we are feeling, our emotions might be anxiety, fear, or panic.

If our alarm continues to sound, getting louder and louder, we might continue up the curve into a state of hypoarousal – a freeze response. This can feel like a state of collapse. We feel unable to cope with the threat or triggers we are faced with. We may feel depressed, powerless, numb, or hopeless. We find ourselves shutting down in response to the alarm and waiting for it to pass. Sometimes the threat will pass, and our stress response curve will begin to come down. Other times, we may find ourselves exposed to chronic levels of threat, and this can have a more significant impact on our bodies. At times that the threat and distress are not reducing or coming down, we can find ourselves flipping between the levels and strategies, helplessly trying to figure out something that will work.

Trauma and the Body

When we have experienced a high level of threat, ideally, we want (like Taylor Swift) to shake it off. This enables us to put the traumatic event we have experienced into the past and bring our usual state of regulation back online. Let's go back to that hungry animal again – we leave our cave to find the hungry animal waiting for us. Our threat response is activated, and we utilise a flight response to run away from the animal. We successfully get away, back into our cave where we are safe, and the animal leaves. We might sit down on the floor and feel our heart racing, our breathing quicker than usual, our skin feeling sweaty, and so on. We might physically shake as our threat response starts to come down – our breathing and heart rate returns to normal, and we know the threat has passed and we are safe again. This is a physiological process of shaking off the threat – moving from our old brain being in the driver's seat where we have responded to danger and back into our new brain controlling the wheel where we feel like our regulated selves again and our whole brain is working together. The threat becomes something that is past, and we can continue in the present.

If the threat response is triggered in the body and we cannot fight or flee the situation, then the trauma can become stuck in the body as we are trapped in the threat. Using our alarm example, this is where the alarm system never turns off completely. The alarm continues in the background. It may be quieter than in the peak of our threat response, but it is constantly there. Using our hungry animal example, this might be when we become trapped inside our caves with the animal just outside the entrance snarling and growling. We can't fight the animal as it is too big and too close, and we can hear other animals coming too. We also can't run (flight) because we are trapped inside the cave. Both our fight and flight responses get stopped and the only option is to collapse. When these responses get stuck in our bodies, we sometimes find we are constantly trying to complete the threat response that has been blocked. When this happens, we can become hyperalert to threat, and we can also find ourselves trying to fight or flee in other ways because we couldn't do that at the time we needed too.

Living with endometriosis was an experience where my threat response was being triggered in my body daily, and I was trapped in that experience. Over the years, I did engage in various threat responses to try to escape it – fighting with professionals to receive care, running away or avoiding the symptoms, avoiding talking about it by saying

I was fine (when I wasn't), and collapsing at home as the daily cycle pushed me to breaking point time and time again.

Prolonged exposure to threat can result in both emotional and physical symptoms including anxiety, depression, fatigue, inability to concentrate, repeated illness/infections, headaches, irritability, poor sleep, disordered eating habits or patterns, and high blood pressure (Schneiderman, Ironson, and Siegel, 2005). It is difficult to know how to begin to gain some control over our bodies when exposure to threat is chronic and feels inescapable. In the final part of this chapter, we will think about ways to connect with our bodies and manage our physiological experience of threat.

Connecting with Threat in Our Bodies

Throughout this book, we have been highlighting the importance of naming our experience to be able to choose how we respond to it (name it to tame it). Below is a recording sheet you can use to bring together your understanding of threat from this chapter and we will then think about our responses to this. I have put in two of my own examples to start you off.

Trigger	Internal/External	Bodily Symptoms	Response
Hospital Appointments	External (the environment, staff) Internal (fear of how I would be treated)	Heart racing Feeling cold – sense of chill Headache	Fight – Irritability or appease – feeling unable to advocate for myself, not speaking up
Smear tests/internal examinations	External (attending the procedure) Internal (pain, physical experience of being examined)	Heart racing Feeling cold – sense of chill Headache	Freeze – feeling disconnected from the experience, finding it difficult to talk to the person

(Continued)

(*Continued*)

Trigger	Internal/External	Bodily Symptoms	Response

As we work together through this book, we are going to think about a range of skills that might enable us to bring compassion to ourselves and our bodies when we are in a state of threat. To achieve this, it can be helpful to develop some skills that address our threat response in a physical way. Simply put, if something is happening in our bodies that has a physical impact on us and makes us feel out of control, we need to do something physically to address it and try to regain some balance.

Mindfulness is a technique that is utilised in CFT as well as other psychological therapies such as cognitive behavioural therapy. Mindfulness focusses on being present in the here and now. I personally found some mindfulness exercises difficult in the context of persistent, severe pain and physical illness. I first tried a mindfulness exercise during a lecture at university. At that time, I was suffering from persistent pain, a common experience in endometriosis. I would go into university wearing heat packs under my clothes and was using strong painkillers throughout the day. During the exercise, we were asked to pay attention to our bodies, turning our attention inwards to ourselves. I remember being completely overwhelmed by this exercise, as when I connected with my body in that moment, all I could focus on was the pain I was trying to ignore. I felt my alarm system getting louder, telling me 'I can't do this, this doesn't feel safe' – I hated connecting with a body that caused me so much distress. I wanted to leave (flight response) and not do the exercise, but I felt unable to do this because I was a student and supposed to be learning from the lecturer's expertise (activating further threat, fear of rejection, shame). I stayed in the lecture and tried to engage with the exercise (please/appease strategy in response to the social threat of being rejected by the lecturer or my peers). However, when we were asked to give our reflections on the exercise, I felt myself being critical of mindfulness and irritable with the lecturer, telling the group I did not see how it could be of any value to anyone (fight response). I went home that day upset and convinced that I would never utilise mindfulness in any form ever again. However, once I learnt about mindfulness from a CFT approach, I was able to reconnect with this and utilise it in a way which was more helpful to me.

Later in this book, we are going to think more about a compassionate approach to persistent pain, including how mindfulness can be applied in a potentially useful way to this. For now, we are going to focus on one of the core skills that underpins the techniques in this book – activating soothing in the body using our breath. We are trying to bring together the two psychologies of compassion we discussed in chapter 4. Turning towards our suffering and distress (by recognising our threat, naming it, knowing it) and having the wisdom to want to change it (by utilising the skills we are developing).

Soothing Rhythm Breathing

As we have identified earlier in this chapter, when our threat response is activated, our breathing can speed up and turn up the volume on our alarm system. This can also cause our heart race to increase. Being able to use soothing rhythm breathing is designed to help manage our threat response, promoting a feeling of calm and safety. It may not turn off the threat response, or remove the trigger, but it may give us more choice of how we respond to the situation we find ourselves in. I found soothing rhythm breathing particularly helpful when sitting in the waiting area for appointments and during physical examinations and procedures. I also remember using this technique when being placed under general anaesthetic.

Soothing rhythm breathing helps to stimulate our parasympathetic nervous system. This can mean keeping the volume of our alarm at a level we can manage, or it may help with turning it down. For me, with the example of physical examinations, it was about keeping the alarm manageable until the examination was over and then continuing to use the rhythm to bring the volume back down.

Trying to breathe in a soothing rhythm can be difficult, but it is not dangerous. Some people find that focussing on their breathing can make them feel more anxious. If this happens to you when you are trying this exercise, please stop and take a break. It might be that you need the support of a clinical psychologist, therapist, or other mental health professional alongside this book in order to develop these skills. The exercise below is adapted from The Compassionate Mind Workbook (Irons and Beaumont, 2017) and is designed to guide you through an example of soothing rhythm breathing. You can also access recordings of exercises like this one on the Compassionate Mind Foundation website.

> *Find a space that allows you to practice engaging with a soothing breathing rhythm. This might be a quiet space, or you may prefer to have some music playing. Find a posture that works for you – usually, you would sit upright with your feet flat on the floor. Bring your back slightly away from the chair so your body is engaged and ready for the exercise. If this way of sitting is uncomfortable or unsuitable for you, you can also try sitting cross-legged on the floor, sitting on the floor with your legs in front of you, or laying down.*
>
> *Place one hand on your chest and another on your tummy – we are going to send your breath down to the hand in your stomach. As you breathe, the hand on your stomach will move, but the one on your chest*

will not. Having your hands on your body can help you to learn how to move your breath through your body in a soothing rhythm. If touching your body or stomach is difficult for you, you might want to sit in front of a mirror and watch the way your body moves. You can also place something on your stomach and use this to monitor your breath – a beanbag is a good option! If this seems too difficult for you, just try paying close attention to the way your breath moves around your body.

Take a breath in through your nose – try to send the air you are breathing in down to that hand on your stomach – filling it up like a balloon. Inhale until you feel comfortably full of air.

Hold the air in your body for two seconds.

Breathe out (this can be through your mouth or nose). You should see the hand on your stomach moving down towards you.

Repeat steps 2–5 at least 5 times (or for around 60 seconds minimum).

When you begin to practice an exercise like this, it is ideal to practice it at times when you are not under high levels of stress. The reality of my experience was there was never a good time to practice it, so find times where you can practice in a manageable way for you. The key to this exercise, like many of the skills in this book, is practicing little and often. I would encourage you to try this a few times throughout the day – my favourite time is when the kettle is boiling. Instead of getting on with other things, try sitting down and breathing in this way for a few minutes. As you practice more, you will become more able to bring this rhythm into your body at times of difficulty.

Summary

- Our threat system can be activated by internal and external triggers. This causes a physical response in our bodies. Our threat system functions to keep us safe, but like the tricky loops in our brain, it can sometimes cause us to feel stuck.

- Being able to recognise our triggers and the physical symptoms threat in our bodies can help us to learn how to respond to this experience and manage it differently.
- Our body has ingrained responses to threat. We cannot turn these responses off as they are there to keep us safe, but we can learn how to manage them and our response to them.
- Traumatic experiences can impact on how we experience threat in our bodies. This might mean we need to take more time to manage our responses and continue to approach ourselves with the qualities of compassion.
- We can learn to connect with our bodies differently to turn down the alarm system and regulate the physical response we are experiencing. Connecting with a soothing breathing rhythm forms the foundation of managing our physical response to threat. Using this skill to bring down our alarm system can help us to then connect with other helpful skills that we will learn later in the book.

6 Understanding Shame and Its Relevance in Endometriosis

What Is Shame?

Shame is an emotion we will all experience at some time in our life. Like threat, it is unavoidable, and the impact shame can have on us differs depending on our response to it. Shame, guilt, and humiliation are central to CFT as these emotions can carry a threat of social disconnection or rejection. Paul Gilbert, the founder of CFT (1998) defines shame as: "*being in the social world as an undesired self: a self one does not wish to be. Shame is an involuntary response to an awareness that one has lost status and is devalued (p.2).*"

Shame can make us feel unworthy or inadequate. The fear of rejection or judgement from others activates our threat system, and this makes us feel vulnerable. Shame is different to guilt. Guilt can be helpful and adaptive as it reminds us that something we have done, or have not done, is not consistent with the kind of person we are or are striving to be. Although this is uncomfortable, it reminds us to modify our behaviour so we can continue to learn and grow. However, shame makes us feel that we are flawed and unworthy of connection (Brené Brown, 2013). Holding onto shame and carrying it around with us is a deep and painful feeling.

If you had asked me to name the emotions I felt in connection with my endometriosis, shame would not have been the first thing I thought of in the past. It took me a long time to understand that I was ashamed, because I was uncomfortable with this feeling. I think of myself as someone who is open and honest, but I was not open with important people in my life about my endometriosis. It is still difficult to be honest about the impact that the illness had on my life and continues to shape how I see my past and future self. You might not identify with shame as part of your experience and choose to skip this chapter. However, I would encourage you to read it to think about whether this does play a role in your life. If it does, beginning to understand, accept, and embrace it can be helpful (it was for me). Brené Brown (2023), a shame and vulnerability researcher, writes 'shame cannot survive being spoken'. This chapter is my attempt to speak to my own experience of shame.

In this chapter, we will think more about shame as a threat (internal and external as discussed in chapter 5), the responses that we use to manage threat and shame, as well as ways to embrace our vulnerabilities and bring compassion to shame.

Why Is Shame a Threat to Us?

Shame makes us feel that we are unacceptable to the group in some way. If we are not accepted by our social groups, we may be rejected or disconnected from others around us. This could mean we are left alone. From an evolutionary perspective, being alone outside of our tribe decreases our chance of survival. It is difficult for a human to survive alone and more beneficial physically and psychologically for us to belong to a group. We are motivated to remain part of the group, and this might mean concealing parts of ourselves from others to prevent the group from excluding us.

Unfortunately, hiding our painful feelings from others can mean we don't use our social groups to their full potential. Our desire to be part of a group is partly because we are very good at cooperating with, and caring for, each other. This helps us to manage our threat responses. Rather than relying on fight, flight, freeze, and please/appease, we can 'care and share' (Gilbert, 2010a). This allows us to turn to others for support, explain how we are feeling, and with support from others we can regulate our emotions differently. Our soothing system is activated, which helps us to manage and reduce our threat response. However, if shame is present, this can get in the way of us seeking this support from others and coping in this way – this may be because 'shame derives its power from being unspeakable' (Brené Brown, 2015). I believe that shame made me feel that my endometriosis was unspeakable to most people in my life and because of that it was powerful, and it left me disconnected, isolated, and afraid.

Where Does Shame Come From and Why Do We Experience Shame?

Like threat, shame can be both internal and external. Shame is a feeling, and like all other feelings it is there to help us. If we can understand shame and its function, then we can socialise ourselves to it rather than become stuck in it. The function of shame is to motivate us to stay within a group. Without it, we might do lots of things that would constantly push us away from others and reduce our chances of survival.

Shame is a painful emotion, and revealing the parts of ourselves that make us feel ashamed to another person can make us feel vulnerable. It can also make us afraid that we won't be met with the compassion and care we need at that moment. Embracing our own vulnerability can trigger all sorts of threat responses in us. Understandably, we often don't want this to happen, and this can mean we avoid revealing shame in lots of different ways. This is one of the challenges of working with shame in therapy – people just don't want to talk about it!

The strategies we use to defend against shame, like many other coping strategies, can have unintended consequences. In trying to keep ourselves safe from rejection, we can sometimes isolate ourselves further as we are unable to share our experience with others, and we do not benefit from the possible 'caring and sharing' that other people can offer. For me, concealing my shame from others extended to healthcare professionals, which impacted on my ability to seek professional support as I felt they would not believe me or respond in a helpful manner.

In CFT, external shame is seen as the central process of shame as our experience of shame often begins on the outside. External shame is where our attention is focussed outside of ourselves, often on the perception others have of us which could result in us being rejected by them. External shame is more strongly associated with anxiety and depression than internal shame. It makes sense that we would want to avoid judgement from others, and we might default to coping strategies that allow us to achieve this such as avoidance. We are trying to choose a response to keep ourselves safe, but the unintended consequence might be losing out on the care and support that others could provide if we could share our experience with them. I think that the stigma associated with periods and endometriosis has an impact on the external shame that can be present for those living with the condition. Always (a company that makes sanitary towels and period products) brought together data from research between 2014 and 2020. This highlights that almost half the people surveyed, across five different countries, felt ashamed or embarrassed about their periods and tried to hide it from others. One in three people had referred to their period as 'gross or disgusting'.

In addition to the external shame and stigma that exists in relation to periods and menstruation, there are additional factors impacting people with endometriosis. At present, it takes an average of eight years to receive a diagnosis of endometriosis (Endometriosis UK, 2023). The All Party Parliamentary Group (2020) found that prior to getting a diagnosis, 58% of women visited their GP more than ten times, 43% visited doctors in hospital over five times, and 53% had visited A&E. Personally, I lost count of how many times I saw a GP or attended hospital, but I was admitted to hospital on approximately five occasions before my diagnosis. Considerable effort is being made at present by dedicated healthcare professionals, organisations, charities, and campaigners to begin to change this. For example, Endometriosis UK are currently campaigning for the UK government to make a commitment to reduce diagnosis time to four years or less by 2025 and a year or less by 2030.

Internal shame is when we begin to believe (internalise) the views of other people, and this can become how we see ourselves. For example, when I first had pain with my periods, I approached other people for help. My mum offered compassion and support, and we went to the school and the GP. Both the teachers and the GP responded by saying it was only a period and that I had a low pain threshold, and it was possible I was overreacting to the pain. I was told by the GP that more exercise would help, and I would get used to it as I grew older. I felt ashamed that I had used the GP's time for something that they didn't think was a problem. This experience happened repeatedly, for many years with different professionals who I feel lacked the knowledge and understanding at that time to realise that my experience might be the result of a gynaecological condition. I was told that I was sensitive, not coping well, not resilient enough, not strong enough, not fit enough, too tall, eating the wrong foods, and exaggerating. This became a strong, consistent message that it was my fault, rather than something was wrong. The repeated message when attempting to access support in my teenage years was that periods were something I had to learn to cope with. When you have enough people say the problem is you, you begin to believe that.

As I continued to receive these messages from external sources, I internalised these beliefs as internal shame. I believed that I was failing to cope, and I was not as strong as other people. I saw myself as weak and inadequate in comparison to others. I believed I was at fault for my suffering – I had lists of things I should have done to help myself, but I couldn't do these things because despite what I believed at the time, my pain and experience was not because I was weak. It was because I had endometriosis and over time, that endometriosis was growing and becoming more severe whereas in my mind, I was becoming weaker and more pathetic.

I know now that I was ashamed. I felt more ashamed over time as I continued to have experiences where I did reach out and I was shamed again by others. I remember being very unwell due to a cyst that had ruptured and become a pelvic infection – this ended up in surgery. My husband had called an ambulance when I collapsed at home – the paramedics came and wanted me to walk down the stairs to the ambulance. I remember saying I couldn't do it – and one of the paramedics tutted and sighed. They told me 'I was going to have to do something because we can't carry you down the stairs'. With the support of my husband, I crawled from my bed and down the stairs, crying and vomiting to the ambulance. The paramedic stood on my driveway, and indiscreetly rolled their eyes at their colleague.

These experiences stopped me from feeling able to seek help and support from others including professionals at times. There are many healthcare professionals and services dedicated to caring for people with endometriosis, but it took me time to reach out to the right services because I had so many difficult experiences in my past. Evidence from Endometriosis UK suggests I am not alone in worrying about access to healthcare support for endometriosis symptoms - 62% of women (aged 16–54) would put off going to a doctor with symptoms of endometriosis because they don't think it's serious enough, they feel embarrassed, or they think their symptoms are normal. I often had to build up my confidence to go to medical appointments or call the GP as I felt I would be faced with this experience again, even though this wasn't the case every time. I did have support from people who loved me and believed that there was something wrong with me, and healthcare professionals who did refer me to the right services and give me the right treatment, but even this support wasn't enough to make my feelings of internal shame go away. I always worried that deep down my family and friends they thought the same as medical professionals or teachers from the past and just weren't being honest with me. This was my new brain adding internal threat to my experience – all the 'what if' thoughts and worries. This internal shame changed the way I saw myself, my relationship with myself and my relationships with other people. I became more critical of myself and punishing, and I found it difficult to trust other people. In chapter 7, we will explore more about how endometriosis and shame can impact our relationship with ourselves and with others and how to bring compassion to these relationships.

I do not want to criticise the medical professionals who I met over the years who did not know how to help me, as endometriosis was not widely recognised at that time. I am also grateful to those who did listen to me and who offered support and compassion. This remains an area of developing research, and information about the disease is growing, so it is understandable that people around me made sense of my symptoms based on the knowledge they had at that time. I also lived in an area without a specialist endometriosis centre, and I didn't know I could access this, or what the difference was between these centres and my local gynaecologist.

There are now changes happening aimed at reducing the stigma, shame, and taboo associated with periods. In 2010, Kotex launched its 'break the cycle' campaign, and in 2017 advertising began to show red blood rather than blue liquid with an aim to normalise menstruation (Bodyform: Blood Normal). Menstrual health education has been made compulsory in schools since 2020 and charities such as the Menstrual Health Project, Period Positive, and Period Poverty UK are all doing outstanding work to change the experience of menstruating people in future.

I support everyone who is currently working to reduce the shame that can be associated with periods, endometriosis, and other gynaecological conditions because this is how we will prevent this cycle from continuing for people like me in the future. I think it is important for us to be able to identify shame, as if we can identify it and name it then shame cannot survive.

Body Shame and Endometriosis

I have talked about the development of shame in terms of my experiences with other people. However, there is a particular type of shame called 'body shame' which I think is important in endometriosis and internal shame that can be associated with living with the illness.

We have talked about how shame is derived from a fear that we are unacceptable to others and might be rejected by them. This might be because of our behaviour or our appearance. Periods and endometriosis are a physical experience, involving our bodies. This can change the way we look, and endometriosis may be associated with physical disability for some of us. I think this is why body shame is important in endometriosis because the illness impacts us in physical ways. Here are some examples from my own experience:

- Fluctuations in weight
- Bloating (this was very significant at times)
- Bleeding (worries about blood being visible on clothing)
- Flare ups of pain sometimes resulting in fainting or vomiting in public
- Disability (not being able to walk as far, stand for long periods, need to use mobility aids at times, etc.).

Some of these symptoms resulted in experiences of body shaming for me, which is a form of bullying where other people make inappropriate or hurtful comments about someone's social appearance (Schluter et al., 2023). I experienced many experiences of body shaming during my journey with endometriosis by many people including strangers, colleagues, and friends. When I was bloated, I was asked if I was pregnant, or people commented on my weight gain. I often used the lift at work due to pain in my legs, and people regularly commented that I didn't need to be using it as I was young or being lazy by doing so. I would always gain weight around my period, and when I attended a slimming club, it would be assumed I hadn't been 'good' that week or had gone off plan. I became very aware of my body and my appearance.

Body shaming, like other kinds of external shame, can become internalised as a perception that our bodies are unattractive or undesirable (Gilbert & Miles, 2002). Body shame can be linked to feelings of self-disgust. This experience for me was most dominant with heavy bleeding. Endometriosis can be associated with heavy periods that last longer than usual. It can also involve bleeding in between periods unexpectedly. My bleeding was very heavy and would last a minimum of ten days. I lost clots of bloods which I found distressing and I often experienced leaks and flooding, where I would bleed through onto my clothes. I did find this disgusting at times (particularly the clots) and I experienced disgust (which activated my threat system) towards me from others. For example, when I was at school, I was bullied because another girl saw a streak of blood on my PE shorts. My threat system was hypervigilant to any feeling that might indicate I was starting to bleed or that bleeding was becoming heavier, as sometimes I would get a gush of blood out of nowhere and usually would need to get to a bathroom quickly to prevent the blood going onto my clothes or the chair where I was sitting. I also worried about sleeping away from home because of getting blood on the sheets. If I did need to sleep away from home during my period, I would be awake most of the night. The threat of the bleeding being noticed by other people, resulting in rejection by them as had happened in my life before, impacted how I saw my period and it became something I was afraid and ashamed of.

My experience of shame resulted in me hiding my experience from others. It made me reluctant to seek help, from anyone including healthcare professionals. It is recognised that in other conditions where body shame is relevant, such as bowel cancer and sexual health, body shame can prevent people from seeking help. I am not aware of specific research looking at body shame and endometriosis, but my experience was one in which I found it difficult to seek help in part due to embarrassment.

I also experienced body shame linked to grief. The progression of the disease meant I experienced a loss of control over my body and its functions over time, and this disconnected me from many things that had helped maintain my self-esteem and connection with others. Every decision seemed to be associated with my endometriosis. I chose clothes that were comfortable, baggy, and dark colours in case of a flare up or bleeding. I kept my hair short because longer hair took energy to maintain, and I didn't have that energy to spare. I was often too exhausted to do things I wanted to or I enjoyed. As my condition worsened, I lost connection with my hobbies – dancing became too painful to bear, I couldn't go to concerts because I couldn't stand up long enough, I lost the passion I had for music and stopped performing. For a long time, I fought to try to maintain these connections by concealing my disability from others, because I did not want to be seen differently by those close to me. It felt like naming what I needed and was going through was a form of giving up. Through using the skills in this book, and with time, I was able to reconnect with some parts of my identity by being open about my needs. However, the grief and the sadness were still there. For example, I joined a choir so I could reconnect with singing again and I enjoyed this. However, to perform I needed to ask for a stool to sit on and explain I couldn't stand for the whole performance. Lots of people then asked why I had the stool, as I did not have a visible disability. For the first time, I was able to say I had endometriosis and pain because of it to relative strangers. Often people would nod in response, but I knew they didn't understand, and I still felt embarrassed. It was a hard change to make but also a first step towards finding the parts of myself I had lost.

In the rest of this chapter, we will think about some of the other external factors that might influence our experience of shame in endometriosis and how we might be able to identify and manage our shame.

Not Naming and Shaming – Naming and Taming!

The first step to understanding our own is shame is understanding that everyone's experience of shame is different. We all grow up in different cultures, generations, social classes, religious/spiritual groups, countries and so on. There are so many things in the world that make our experiences unique, and shame is no different – it is not the same for everyone.

It can be helpful to start thinking about your own experience of shame in terms of what you have learnt is (or isn't) acceptable to your group from the people, culture, and world around you. We begin to develop a sense of how things 'should' or 'shouldn't' be from the world around us, including the way we look, behave, the opinions we have and so on. Another way to think about your worldview is what you mean when you say or think of something as 'normal'. Normal means it is what is typical or expected to you, based on your experience, but we also know that what is normal for you might not be normal for me.

This can apply to a huge range of things; some are small and might be less shameful to us and others might be very big. A small example might be like this – I don't think you *should* have mushy peas with a roast dinner. However, my husband's family often have mushy peas with Sunday Lunch. This was completely outside my 'normal' for what you eat with Sunday Lunch – I exclaimed that it was a weird side dish, and I didn't eat it! In this situation, my in-laws laughed, and I don't think were ashamed about their decision to eat mushy peas with roast beef. However, they were the majority – they had a social group they belonged to who all ate mushy peas. As the minority, I knew that this social group was not going to reject me for not eating the peas, so I was free from shame and able to give my true opinion. Although there is difference of opinion here as to what is 'normal' or how a roast dinner 'should' look, it wasn't going to lead to rejection from the group for any of us, so we could all laugh about it and still enjoy our family meal.

Understanding Shame and Its Relevance in Endometriosis

Sometimes our expectations of how things should be and what is normal are much bigger than this. This can then impact how we feel about ourselves and we can feel worried or afraid that if we are not doing things the way we believe we should, other people will not want to be around us, and we will be left alone. In chapter 2, we talked about how menstrual education may contribute to our views of periods and how we should manage them. For me, this developed some of the 'shoulds' around periods that I carried as shameful throughout my life.

One way to identify possible places of shame in your own life is to starting spotting shoulds. If you look back through this chapter, you will notice quite a few! Shoulds can become problematic when they become rules. When shoulds become rules, they can carry a lot of power in our lives and leave us feeling inadequate, like a failure or ashamed.

I learnt a lot of shoulds about periods and symptoms of endometriosis during my life. I have put together a top five on the left. On the right, is a space for you to add any shoulds you have which might be the same or different to mine.

Shoulds	
<ul><li>I should be able to cope with my period pain.</li><li>I should be able to carry on with my normal life during my period.</li><li>I should avoid talking to other people about my period.</li><li>I should exercise during my period.</li><li>I should keep my period secret from other people.</li></ul>	

As you notice your shoulds, you might begin to make connections with feelings of shame or self-criticism. Here is an exercise for you to begin to identify and challenge your shoulds.

EXERCISE – Shifting your should

Question	My Example	Your Example
Whose should is this? Where did it come from?	I should exercise during my period. I learnt this at school and from other resources which promote gentle exercise during your period.	
Does this should help me? Do I want this should? If not, send it back to where it came from – let it go. Some people like to send back unwanted shoulds in visual ways – writing them down and throwing them away, visualising them disappear, saying them out loud and letting them go can all be used to send back the should if you feel that is helpful to you.	The idea I should exercise during my period increased my suffering, because I would push myself to try to go for a walk when I was in severe pain. At its worst, this resulted in fainting. However, I had been told that I should be able to do this, and it would make things better. I believed that not doing this meant I was weak, so I pushed myself too hard. When you are in severe pain due to endometriosis, exercise is often impossible. I needed to let go of the idea that this was something I should do.	
What happens if you change this should to a could? If you change some of your shoulds to coulds, how does this change what you are thinking or feeling?	Could I exercise during my period? – for me, the answer to this question was clear. I often struggled to walk to the toilet. Exercise was not manageable for me during these times. However, at other times in my cycle, I benefited from a walk, yoga, and dancing. I found that when I used could, it felt like I have a choice rather than a rule/must. I found it helpful to remind myself, if I could do this, I would, and I noticed that when I could connect with exercise in a helpful way, I was doing this more often than I had realised.	

(*Continued*)

(*Continued*)

Question	My Example	Your Example
Can you change the should to a would like? Does this change what you are thinking or feeling?	I would like to do gentle exercise during my period. This is true – I wanted to be able to do more during my period. Not necessarily exercise (I can't imagine ever being an athlete!), but I would like to be able to walk my dog or go around the shops. It might be that this is not possible because of the severity of symptoms, and we may need to bring some compassion to ourselves in that (see chapter 7). Alternatively, it might be that there are things we can do to work towards the way we would like things to be.	

Now you have experimented with different ways of shifting your shoulds, try to choose a replacement for the should that feels more helpful to you. Sometimes I found 'I could' statements difficult because sometimes I felt angry; they were untrue in that moment. For example, I could not exercise if I could barely walk. However, I would like to statements felt less threatening in these situations. Sometimes I found the best thing for me was just to let go of the should statement completely because the alternatives did not quite fit with my experience at the time. Remember this is about finding what works for you, so feel free to explore the ideas that you find helpful and leave the ones you do not.

Naming Shame in Ourselves

Another way to begin to identify shame is to think about how we feel physically and emotionally when we are experiencing it. We can draw on our learning from chapter 5 on how we identify physical feelings associated with threat in our body, as shame is a form of threat – the threat of social rejection.

You might want to look back at the exercise in chapter 5 where you identified how threat feels in your body. This might help you to think about the bodily feelings that might come up when you experience shame. There might also be certain thoughts or emotions that come up at these times too, which you can add into this worksheet.

My Example	Your Example
When I feel shame, my threat system responds with physical symptoms in my body. I feel / It feels like: *a shiver in my body, a sensation of my heart stopping like when I hit the brakes on a car. I can feel the adrenaline rush through my body, which makes my heart rate increase and I breathe faster. I feel my senses sharpen as I become hyper alert to what is happening around me. It can also feel like I am smaller and I want to hide away.*	When I feel shame, my threat system responds with physical symptoms in my body. I feel / It feels like:
I know I am in shame when I feel: *less than others, embarrassed, quiet/withdrawn, powerless, and silenced.*	I know I am in shame when I feel:
I want to be perceived as / do not want to be perceived as: *I want to be perceived as strong, resilient, and able to cope. I do not want to be perceived as weak, pathetic, or disgusting.*	I want to be perceived as / do not want to be perceived as:

Once you have identified these physical sensations in your body, you might want to think back to the strategies in chapter 5 to manage physical threat in our bodies. You can apply these skills whenever you notice the symptoms associated with threat in your body. Below, you might want to bullet-point what is helpful for you:

> When I am experiencing physical symptoms of threat, it is helpful for me to…..

Bringing Compassion to Shame

Now that we understand what shame is and where it might be present in our lives, let's turn our attention to thinking about the ways we can bring compassion to shame. Shame is linked to threat and this can block our connection to others. To bring compassion to shame, we need to be able to notice it, name it, and understand it. This is what we have worked on in this chapter. The other part of managing our shame is being able to turn towards it with compassion. In chapters 7 and 8, we are going to work on developing our compassionate self and compassionate other so you can connect with compassion at times of challenge. As we build on these skills, remember to continue working on the soothing rhythm breathing that we covered in chapter 5, as this is the foundation for the exercises we will develop as we move through the book.

Summary

- Shame is a difficult and painful emotion. Shame makes us feel we are unacceptable to the group, and this can make us feel disconnected from others. Sometimes we might also disconnect

- from others or avoid sharing our experience with others because we fear being rejected by them.
- Shame can be both external and internal. External shame comes from those around us, or fears of how we might be perceived by others. Internal shame is when we begin to internalise the views of others, and this can become how we see ourselves.
- There is a type of shame called body shame and this is relevant in endometriosis because of the impact the condition has on our bodies. This body shame can also be internalised and impact our relationships with our bodies and ourselves.
- The first step in tackling shame is naming and taming! This is because shame cannot survive being spoken (Brene Brown).
- We can also work to bring compassion to our shame using the later skills in this book.

7 Endometriosis and Your Relationship with Yourself

In chapter 6, we talked about the shame and its relevance to endometriosis. We considered both external and internal shame. In this chapter, we will think more about internal shame and how this can manifest as internal self-criticism or self-hatred. Self-criticism is very common, particularly in Western cultures (Irons and Beaumont, 2017), and can keep us caught up in threat. As we have learnt earlier in this book, there are also specific components of living with endometriosis that might contribute to internal shame and self-criticism.

Internal shame can sometimes be present in the way we talk to ourselves. Although talking to yourself is not always seen as a positive thing, it is something that we all do, all the time. Some of us might do this aloud, and we will all do this internally. This internal self-talk is there to help motivate us, make sense of things, make decisions, and keep us moving forward in our lives. When this is working well, it is very helpful – lots of long-distance runners refer to this inner talk as aiding them in making it over the finish line. However, when our inner self-talk is critical, this can be painful and damaging. CFT refers to this internal voice saying unkind and judgemental things to yourself as the self-critic.

So why do we do it? For the same reasons that we find ourselves caught in other tricky loops, because as humans we often can't help it. Like many of the other threat-based experiences we have discussed in this book, the self-critic has a function. It is there to try to help us in some way. For example, if we are worried about what outfit to choose for an important event and the critic is telling us the outfit isn't right or doesn't look good, it might be trying to remind us that this event is very important to us, we might be feeling nervous about the event and finding an outfit we are comfortable in makes us feel more confident about attending. It can help to understand the motives of our self-critic, so we can bring compassion towards it.

Understanding Your Own Self-Criticism and Self-Critic

Our self-criticism can be focussed on almost anything about ourselves that we feel we do not like or that we perceive others do not like about us. This might be our physical appearance, our personality, our attributes, or our behaviour. Much of my self-criticism focussed on factors associated with my endometriosis, but there were other parts of my personality, skills, and identity that did not carry the same self-criticism or internal shame. Sometimes self-criticism might still show up for me in these areas, but crucially, it did not cause me distress. In this chapter, we are thinking about self-criticism that causes us distress. This distress might be feeling that we are not good enough or disgusting. We might even feel destructive towards ourselves. When this happens, we might have a desire to punish ourselves for our failures which can lead to unhelpful and even harmful behaviours.

One of the techniques CFT uses to help us understand our self-criticism is imagery. Later in this chapter, there is an exercise to help you imagine your own self-critic. I found it helpful to think about my self-criticism as coming from an self-critic inside me (I sometimes called this an inner critic), a little part of myself that was well-intentioned but often triggered tricky loops for me. This helped me to notice it, name it, and begin to relate to it with more compassion and understanding.

When we begin to try to understand our own self-criticism, we may first want to think about the things from our past which might have contributed to this. This may link to some of the background factors in the four-part formulation you completed in chapter 4. There are several factors that can influence the development of self-criticism. This can include the kinds of relationships we have had in the past with other people, our life experiences, and social media.

If we have had relationships with people who were critical towards us, we may internalise this and be more critical of ourselves. Your self-critic may even say things that others in your life have said to you before. For those of us who have experienced traumatic events in our life, or significant challenges, this can be another trigger for self-critical thoughts. In addition, there is now increasing evidence that messages from the media, including social media, which tell us how we should look, what we should have, and how we should feel and behave can also contribute to feelings of shame and self-criticism (Irons and Beaumont, 2017). My self-criticism developed in part, due to multiple experiences with other people that developed and then reinforced negative beliefs about myself. I experienced many conversations with healthcare professionals which made me feel misunderstood and invalidated, and I often felt friends and family couldn't understand my experience even if this wasn't their intention. I had also experienced bullying from others at school which impacted the way I saw myself. You may also have experienced rejection or even cruelty from others in response to your symptoms. This may have impacted the way in which you seek support from others (see chapter 7) and the way you talk and relate to yourself.

As we have discussed throughout this book, our three systems have a function and self-criticism is no different. Our self-criticism may have several functions. It may be trying to motivate us, thinking that if it is hard on us this will make us act in a certain way. Our self-critic may also want us to feel in control, so it can tell us had we behaved differently, then the outcome might be different. However, this is not always the case. For example, my self-critic tells me that if I had fought earlier on in my journey for treatment and diagnosis maybe my endometriosis would not have become as severe as it did (another example I believed proved I was weak and pathetic for not fighting harder for my own health and well-being). Although accessing different treatment at different times might have changed my journey in some way, it is unlikely that anything I did would have stopped or prevented the progression of an incurable disease. However, admitting how little control we have over our lives can be scary, and it might feel easier to blame ourselves. The self-critic might also be trying to keep us safe as self-criticism activates the brain's threat response. Unfortunately, if we see the threat as ourselves, self-criticism doesn't work well. Our old brain is triggered and can attack us increasing our critical self-talk.

Imagining the Self-Critic

I find it helpful to have an image of my self-critic in my mind. This has helped me to understand my self-criticism as coming from a part of me that is trying to help but does not always succeed. As a clinical psychologist, I have worked with other people who have also found it helpful to imagine their self-critic. I have known people create visual examples of their critic through drawing or collage which has been helpful to them. I see my self-critic as a little fuzzy monster – I think this is because of a cartoon I saw as a child where the character had a little monster inside that made the character grumpy! I associate my self-criticism with a darkness that at its worst makes me feel cold and anxious. It speaks like a strict teacher making me feel small and insignificant. It is gender-fluid depending on what it says to me at the time, sometimes it will sound more male and sometimes more female. It rarely shouts, but always speaks with authority. Sometimes it speaks with mild disapproval which I find easier to cope with, other times it is more powerful, and I have to work harder to manage it.

> *You might want to take some time here to draw, imagine, or write about your self-critic. Have a think about what your critic might look like and sound like? Is it human or non-human? Does it have a form or is it more fluid? How does it speak to you and what emotion does*

it direct towards you? How does it make you feel to be in the presence of this critic? What does it look like, sound like, feel like to be around?

If you have been able to imagine your self-critic, what have you learnt from this? How might this help you to approach it differently?

_____
_____
_____
_____

Now that you have an image of your critic in your mind, we will think about when your self-critic shows up for you and where it focusses its attention. My self-criticism focussed on a range of things including my appearance ('I am unattractive'), my physical limitations ('I am lazy'), and my response to pain ('I am weak for not coping with this pain'). These statements and words made me feel distressed and disconnected. I wondered why I was being so hard on myself when there was a part of me, and people around me, saying different things with more compassion to these statements that I kept repeating in my head.

You may find that you are already able to identify your own self-criticism, but this can also be difficult at first. It took me time to recognise that I was being critical of myself, because I misunderstood the function of the self-criticism as drive based and there to help me to keep going rather than seeing this was threat based drive and how it maintained threat for me and could lead to collapse. You might want to spend some time filling out the table below to bring your awareness to your self-criticism and how it makes you feel. I have put in an example from my own experience which may or may not be helpful for you. Remember that not all self-criticism causes distress, which may mean it is not a problem for you, but you may notice areas that your criticism does cause you to feel upset or unhappy. It might be these areas you want to focus on bringing compassion to later in this chapter.

Situation: What happened when I noticed self-criticism show up for me?	What did I say to myself in this moment?	What do I think the function of this self-criticism might have been?	How did that make me feel? What impact did it have on me?
Booking a GP appointment and being asked if it was urgent as the doctors were very busy today	*You are wasting people's time – this is not urgent or an emergency.* *Why can't you cope with a simple period.* *They have already told you there's nothing wrong – what do you expect from ringing them again? This is your fault for not being able to manage pain.*	*To punish myself by not seeking help because I believed I did not deserve it.*	*Ashamed, guilty, hopeless, and worthless.*

In the first part of this chapter, we have begun to understand our self-criticism and imagine our self-critic. Now that we have this understanding, we want to be able to work on bringing compassion to our self-criticism. As we know, we cannot make our self-criticism go away because it is there for a reason and has a role to play in our lives. However, we want to be able to work on reducing the distress that might be present for us because of it. Changing how we relate to ourselves does not change the symptoms of endometriosis, but I found that it did help me to reduce the psychological impact that the symptoms had on me and my life.

Developing a Compassionate Self

As we have identified in this chapter, many of us have a self-critic that might activate our threat system. CFT helps us to develop a compassionate self (like a compassionate other from chapter 7). For me, I found it helpful to think about both my self-critic and my compassionate self as a part of my identity. CFT recognises that we are all made up of multiple versions of ourselves. When we first think about this, we may get confused in thinking about different parts of our identity such as wife, mother, clinical psychologist, friend, and so on. Although endometriosis can impact our identity, the idea of multiple selves in CFT relates more to parts of us that exist in the same moment but may behave differently to each other. For example, when you are told by a healthcare professional that your symptoms are normal, there might be a part of you that is angry and wants to shout at them and tell them they are wrong. Another part of you might feel anxious that if this person doesn't understand, maybe no one will understand and maybe will never get better. Another part might be sad and hopeless and want to hide away. It is a moment where different feelings are all showing up at once. Using our compassionate selves can help us to connect with these different feelings and responses without shame or judgement.

To achieve this connection in that moment, you need to be able to connect with a wise, strong, kind compassionate self that can tolerate the professional we are talking to not knowing how to help us and be committed to continue to assert ourselves and move towards finding a solution to the problem we are facing. When we begin to develop a compassionate self, it can be helpful to return to the key qualities of compassion which we outlined in chapter 4. Take a moment to think about the key qualities that your compassionate self might need to be able to help you at times of challenge. It might be helpful to break these down into three key areas which we know are helpful when developing a compassionate self.

1. Wisdom: It is important that we can apply wisdom to the challenges we face in life. Wisdom in CFT includes the acceptance that we will all experience pain and difficulties in life, but it also allows us to step back and consider what we can do to alleviate or reduce our distress associated with those difficulties. For me, the wisdom from my compassionate self often helped me to stay out of a tricky loop I named 'why me', where I could get caught up in feeling my experience was unjust or unfair.
2. Caring-Commitment: Compassion is about the genuine desire to care for a person who is suffering. We can be kind without really connecting with this genuine feeling of compassion. Building a compassionate mind involves the commitment to alleviate the distress experienced by other people and by ourselves. It includes the recognition that the difficulties we are experiencing are not our fault, but rather than avoiding these difficulties, we can turn towards them. I have learnt that sometimes bringing my compassionate self to my struggles means still doing something that is challenging for me (see compassionate behaviour: chapter 9) but approaching this from a different position, which reduces my distress.
3. Strength and Courage: Being compassionate to other people and/or ourselves means that we are willing to connect with distress. This can make us feel vulnerable and activate threat for us. In chapter 9, we will think about persistent pain and how difficult it can be to turn towards this pain when it might be easier to try to avoid it. Connecting with distress requires us to connect with inner strength and courage so we can engage with the feelings and sensations without becoming overwhelmed. Strength and courage are the foundations of the compassionate life we want to build for ourselves.

There is no right or wrong way to develop your compassionate self – different people find different things work for them, so I am going to give you a few different ideas in this chapter. Developing a compassionate self is not an easy thing to do, and you might find that yours evolves over time as you practice these exercises. Sometimes people find a guided exercise a good place to start. This exercise is adapted from

The Compassionate Mind Workbook (Irons and Beaumont, 2017). Remember to find a comfortable position before starting this exercise. If an upright sitting position isn't suitable for you, feel free to adjust the positioning to something that works for you but remember to stay actively engaged with the exercise.

> *Take a few moments to connect with your breathing and when you are ready, engage a soothing rhythm to your breath. Relax your face and body.*
>
> *Now, we are going to create a character. This character is going to be of a compassionate person, and you are going to try to act like this character, as if you are an actor taking on this role in a play or a film. You don't have to be this person, just act like them.*
>
> *This character is your compassionate self. It embodies the three qualities of compassion – wisdom, strength, and caring-commitment.*
>
> *First, wisdom. Your compassionate self knows that wisdom comes from many places. They understand that we all have brains that can get caught up in tricky loops. This is not our fault. We didn't choose this brain, and we may not have chosen many other things in our lives that shape us. We didn't choose our genes, gender, ethnicity, or our culture. Nor did we choose to have endometriosis or problems with our health, and yet all these things have a significant impact on who we become.*
>
> *The wisdom of your compassionate self (this character we are creating) is also supporting you to learn how to take responsibility to*

do something about your suffering. This means stepping away from blame, shame, and criticism and focussing our minds in ways that will be helpful. They are helping you to understand that if this version of you is not how you would like it to be, then you can do something about this. Take a few breaths here whilst you take on the role of this wise, compassionate person.

Next let's think about the strength and confidence this character brings. They are like a tree, with deep roots that remains standing through a storm. Like the tree, your compassionate self can be rooted in the presence of distress and not be overwhelmed. Take a moment to focus on the strength of your compassionate self, holding its posture in the face of stress in life. You might want to adapt your posture to suit the role of your compassionate self.

Lastly, let's focus on the deep caring-commitment your compassionate self holds for you. It is wise and recognises life is hard. It wants to do everything it can to reduce your distress. Imagine this part of yourself has an energy, driving it forward to do everything it can to support you and help you.

Try to imagine the qualities of wisdom, strength, and caring-commitment coming together into a sense of your compassionate self. Try to connect with this version of yourself, focussing on the different qualities and the intention of the compassionate self towards you and other people.

When you are ready, allow the image and feeling of your compassionate self to fade and focus your attention back to your soothing rhythm

> *breathing, your body and your surroundings. When you are ready, gently open your eyes.*

There is a space below for you to note down any thoughts you have about your compassionate self or to draw something that has come to mind during this exercise.

> *If you have been able to imagine your compassionate self, what have you learnt from this? How might this help you to approach the multiple parts of yourself, including your self-critic, differently?*

_____
_____
_____
_____
_____

My compassionate self doesn't have a form or a face. It is associated with lightness, both in terms of physical light unlike the dark of my critic and also a feeling of lightness. It feels like the part of me that goes 'ahhh' and releases some of the tension I hold when I'm in threat. It connects me to the soothing rhythm breathing we learnt in chapter 5. It talks to me in the way I talk to other people I love and care about. Unlike my gender-fluid self-critic, my compassionate self is always the voice of a woman.

The important thing in developing your compassionate self is that you can bring to mind a person, character or version or yourself, that embodies compassion.

Connecting with the Self-to-Self Flow of Compassion

Throughout the book, we have talked about the flows of compassion. Self-compassion is when we are directing the flow of compassion from self-to-self. For some of us, it feels difficult to be compassionate to ourselves even if we find it easy to be compassionate to others. If you think back to the exercise in chapter 3, you may have find it easier to offer compassion to me than you would have done to offer it to yourself. This is because we sometimes treat ourselves in ways we would not treat other people. Our self-critic might show up with a loud voice and an imposing presence and overwhelm us. It can take time to connect with our compassionate selves and the flow of self-to-self compassion.

Now you have developed a compassionate self, you can begin to use this to think about connecting with compassion for yourself at times of challenge. This can be done in lots of ways including compassionate self-talk, focussing compassion on yourself, and compassionate behaviour. Let's think about each of these ideas here.

Several practices in CFT ask you to direct intentions, hopes, and feelings towards yourself. Some of the exercises in CFT give you a statement in the exercise, such as may you be well, and you can repeat this statement. I found it helpful to make my own versions of these statements that worked best for me. Some people call these mantras or positive affirmations. I call them coping statements, and I find it helpful to use the same ones repeatedly. When you consider that our self-critic often repeats the same criticisms to us, or that our self-criticism can follow a theme, it makes sense (at least to me!) that we might use self-compassion in the same way.

Below are some examples of intentions, affirmations, and coping statements from CFT that might inspire you, as well as some of my own examples. In the third column, you may want to add in your own. I have found that these often have the most impact when you can connect with them, at least some of the time. For example, I found it hard when exercises would give statements such as 'may you be well' as my critic would jump in 'I'm not well though am I?'. Whereas a statement such as 'I am strong' felt truer for me – sometimes it didn't feel very true at all, but that was when I needed my compassionate self to remind me that it was true more often than it was false.

My Examples	Other Examples	Your Examples
I am strong	I am enough	
It is OK that this is difficult for me and for me to express that to other people	I am worthy of kindness and compassion	
I can survive this challenge; I have survived many challenges in the past	I matter	
I will embrace my full self, including the parts that make me feel vulnerable, as they are what make me stronger	I do my best, and my best is good enough	
	I am resilient	
	I am brave	

Once you have your statements, you may want to try using them to bring compassion to yourself in this exercise. This is an exercise you can also use anytime. I often used this before hospital appointments, admissions, or surgery which were often high-threat experiences for me.

> *Begin with your soothing rhythm breathing, relaxing your face and body. Bring into your mind the character we created earlier, your compassionate self. You might imagine how they look, or think about the qualities they have, and how it feels to be around them.*
>
> *Remember your compassionate self wants to support you with genuine kindness. Repeat your coping statements to yourself. Notice how it feels to direct these to yourself with warmth and kindness. Repeat these statements as many times as is helpful for you.*

Note down any thoughts, feelings, or reflections you have on the exercise here.

_____
_____
_____
_____

When you begin practising using these coping statements, you might want to take the time to complete this exercise in full. This is because it brings together imaging your compassionate self with connecting with these statements. However, over time, you may find that reminding yourself of these statements is enough to reduce your distress. You can also use these statements in the next exercise, as part of compassionate self-correction.

Compassionate Self-Correction

As we have acknowledged, beginning to be more compassionate to ourselves does not make our self-critic, or self-criticism, go away. However, it may allow us to reduce the threat that we feel in our body and in our mind. We have focussed on shame and threat, whilst knowing the antidote to both is compassionate and connection. In this chapter, we have thought about bringing more compassion to ourselves, and in the next chapter, we will think about connection with compassion from others.

Although I am now free from many of the physical symptoms associated with my endometriosis, when my remaining symptoms show up, so does my self-critic. However, I now expect their arrival and anticipate their behaviour so I can prepare for this (see compassionate behaviour, chapter 9 and below), and I can self-correct when I notice myself falling back into threat. As we have covered, the self critic is trying to be helpful but approaches us in a way which is often unhelpful. If we can keep the intention of the critic, but with a compassionate stance, this enables us to turn towards our difficulties and motivates us to keep working on them. Being compassionate to ourselves is not about making excuses (which I often believed in the past), it is about helping us to manage our distress differently.

As you notice your self-criticism, try countering it with some compassionate self-correction. Here are some examples:

Trigger/situation	Self-criticism	Feelings	Compassionate self-correction	Any change in feeling?
Going to the doctor and leaving with no treatment plan	See, there is nothing wrong with you. You are over-reacting. If the doctor doesn't believe you, no one else will either.	Sad, ashamed, angry	It's understandable I am disappointed and upset that this appointment was not helpful. I know that not all appointments will be like this and other people have been more understanding of what is happening for me. It's not my fault this appointment did not go the way I had hoped. Although it is difficult for me, I am going to call back again and ask for another appointment with a different doctor to get my voice heard. I can also speak to others about what has happened so they can support me next time.	

In chapter 7, we have thought about how endometriosis impacts our relationship with ourselves, and we have begun working on developing our self-to-self flow of compassion using our compassionate self. In chapter 8, we will look at how endometriosis can impact our connection with others and how we can connect with the other-self flow of compassion.

Summary

- When shame becomes internalised, this can become internal self-criticism. In CFT this is called the self-critic.
- Understanding our self-critic can help us to be compassionate towards it and reduce some of the distress it causes us. We can think about the focus of our self-critic, the content of what it says to us, its function, and its origin to help improve our understanding of it. Imagining the self-critic can also be helpful as we learn to approach it differently.
- To balance our self-critic, it can be helpful to have a compassionate self. The role of the compassionate self is not to argue with the critic or try to win, but to connect with compassion towards the critic and direct the flow of compassion from the compassionate part of ourselves to the critical part. This is self-to-self compassion through connecting with multiple parts of ourselves.
- Developing a compassionate self can be done in lots of ways. There is no right or wrong way of doing this; it is important to find the approach that feels right for you.
- Once you have developed your compassionate self, you can work on bringing this part of you to your struggles. Like all of the skills we are learning in this book, this takes practice and time.

8 Endometriosis and Relationships

How Endometriosis Impacts Relationships

In chapter 6, we talked about how shame can be triggered by those around us and how it can be internalised and impact our identity. For me, this impacted my relationships with other people and my relationship with myself. When I felt shame, I would try to move away from it and avoid it. This was a safety strategy (see four-part formulation in chapter 3) with the unintended consequence of disconnecting me from others around me and at times making me feel very alone. I also feel that many situations were more difficult for me because I found it hard to share my difficulties with others. This may have contributed to further trauma as I was not able to access the care and support from others, including specialist healthcare professionals, that may have helped me at times of challenge.

I had symptoms of endometriosis from around 13–14 years of age. For many years, I did not know how to explain my experience to other people, and I would avoid talking about it as much as possible. If I did need to give some information about it to someone, I would usually refer to problems with my periods or a symptom of the condition that felt easier to explain or more socially acceptable to others. For years of my life, people thought I suffered from severe back pain (which was partly true, but not completely). When I did have an understanding that my difficulties, including my back pain, were likely to be endometriosis, I started to name this to other people. This felt like a huge step, but I felt anxious about calling it endometriosis when I did not have a confirmed diagnosis. It made me feel like I was lying because I did not know for sure. Also, when I did name my symptoms as likely to be the result of endometriosis, sometimes this disclosure was not received in the way I wanted or needed. Most people did not know what it was and if they did, they did not understand the impact it can have and was having on me. This sometimes made me feel invalidated and misunderstood by others. However, as awareness of endometriosis improves my experience of sharing my diagnosis with others has changed, and I hope it will be better for other people talking about their diagnosis in the future.

In every significant relationship in my life, there was a moment when I needed to decide whether I would disclose my endometriosis and the impact it was having on me. This applied to friendships, romantic relationships, colleagues, managers, and family members. My overwhelming experience of trying to talk to other people about my endometriosis was that they did not understand. Even people closest to me sometimes gave responses that made me feel dismissed and misunderstood, an experience that is recognised within the literature (Young et al., 2014). I often felt that people thought I was exaggerating my symptoms, even when I felt I was downplaying them. My husband, the most supportive person in my life, has said that seeing the difference in me since my hysterectomy and excision surgery has made him reflect that he did not fully appreciate how disabled I was by my endometriosis. This is one of the many challenges with endometriosis; it is difficult to believe that the person telling you about their experience really does feel this way, because they often appear functional and OK. I know now that my husband, and other people close to me, may not always have understood that my symptoms were as severe as I am now discussing because I did not show that to them. In fact, I worked very hard to hide it. I do not blame the people in my life for perhaps questioning my experience, but it has made me consider how difficult it is to speak openly about endometriosis to people who may never fully understand. I think for this reason endometriosis carries a double threat burden, as it is a physical threat to us and can also cause social disconnection, a further threat. These together made my experience particularly difficult to manage.

In the later stages of my disease, as I considered treatment options, I began to use online support groups and message boards to find out more about the illness and the choices available to me. These were invaluable in gaining information to allow me to make an informed choice about my treatment options. However, I continued to avoid talking to anyone else with endometriosis for peer support because I still felt like an imposter. The impact of my endometriosis was very variable, and I felt they were people more impacted by the disease than I was; therefore, I felt it was not fair for me to speak about my illness when 'it could be worse'. Even in writing this book, I continue to worry about whether my experience will be 'good enough' to justify sharing it and about what other people will think of the choices I have made. However, I also believe that being able to openly talk about my experience is empowering and gives back some control. I think it activates my drive system in a healthier way. This book is an example of drive where I have wanted to produce something that might make a difference to other people. Talking about endometriosis and its impact has been very difficult for me throughout my life, so sharing it openly here has been a challenging experience. Sharing your experience may also be difficult for you, perhaps for the many reasons we have discussed so far. Through my own journey, I have been able to connect with the support and compassion from other people, including friends, families, healthcare professionals and other people with endometriosis. I also know that there were many times I tried to reach out to others for support, and this was not met with compassion. Every time you embrace your vulnerability and reach out to another person, you take a risk, because we never know exactly how that person will respond. Although I came to believe that everyone would respond negatively to me, and this made me avoid connection, I have since learnt that this is not, and was not always, true. As attitudes towards menstrual health and endometriosis continue to change and be challenged, I hope that it will become easier for you and others to share your experiences in future and that these disclosures are more likely to be met with compassion and understanding.

In this chapter, I will share a little about how endometriosis impacted different relationships in my life. I did not find it easy to speak about my illness in any of my relationships. As we have discussed in previous chapters, this was, in part, because of my experience of shame and stigma associated with the disease. I did not know how to begin these conversations with other people, and I noticed that when I felt I was being open about my experience, it was not received in the way I expected. Think back to chapter 6; we are not naming and shaming in disclosure, we are naming and taming so we can care and share with others, activating our soothing systems and responding to threat differently.

Endometriosis at Work

As discussed in chapter 1, I wanted to be a clinical psychologist since I was a teenager. I knew it was a competitive area, and I spent a lot of time in my drive system, focussing on the goal of qualifying as a clinical psychologist. After I completed my undergraduate degree, I was successful in getting my first full-time job as an assistant psychologist. I was so focused on succeeding in this job that I lost sight of taking care of my own health and making the adjustments needed to manage the symptoms I had at that time. This was my pattern, of threat based drive. When this happened, I would disconnect and avoid the symptoms, the shame, and my emotion until my body would force me to connect due to flare ups, severe and persistent pain, or fatigue. This resulted in one of the recurrent urine infections I had turning into a kidney infection which then turned into urosepsis. I remember going to work and sitting through a training day with a high fever, nausea, and dizzy spells. I collapsed when I returned home and was admitted to the hospital that evening. This was one of the most serious hospital admissions of my life. I spent time in the high-dependency unit due to sepsis and I was life-threateningly unwell. When I was admitted to the hospital, I remember worrying about work. I worried that my manager would perceive my sickness as a weakness, and I would not be supported to return to work or to apply for clinical training. When I came out of the hospital, I pushed myself to go back to work as soon as possible and my pattern of threat based drive continued.

The threat of losing my professional identity and career has carried with me throughout my life. In part, this has also been driven by the threat of external shame from others and a worry about rejection from my employers and respected colleagues. Like other relationships in my life, my relationship with work was one where I would avoid disclosure and try to keep my difficulties a secret from my employers due to fears that I would lose my job or that I would be perceived as not good enough at work. According to research by BUPA (2023), I am not alone in worrying about how endometriosis would impact my work and career. 40% of women with endometriosis worry about losing their job, 27% have missed out on a promotion because of their endometriosis, 54% feel endometriosis has reduced their income, and 87% think it has impacted their long-term financial situation. One in six women give up work due to the condition, and 55% 'often' have had to take time off work because of their symptoms

When I reflect now on how I managed my endometriosis at work, I kept many things secret from my managers and colleagues, and I think this was unhelpful at times. At the time, I believed I was using a 'need-to-know' approach to disclosure at work, meaning I would tell managers when there was a specific need to do so. The problem here was my definition of 'need-to-know', which meant I would only tell them if it was completely unavoidable. This made it less of a decision to seek help and support and more being forced into giving them some information which I often kept as minimal as possible, for example, saying I have a hospital appointment but not discussing why. However, as a manager now myself, I would define 'need-to-know' very differently as if there is something work can do to help you, then they need to know so they can help and support. Even if there is nothing they can practically do, it can also sometimes be helpful to know what you are experiencing so that they have some understanding. There were many things that would have helped me at work that I did not access or even know existed because of my definition of 'need-to-know'. This included workplace equipment that would have made my work station more comfortable and may have reduced my pain, flexible working arrangements to manage fatigue and hospital appointments, occupational health support to look at workplace adjustments in managing the condition and home-working arrangements. In chapter 2, we talked about the definition of disability under The Equality Act (2010). This is also something you can discuss with your employers and you may be able to use schemes such as access to work in the UK. I think at times it might have been helpful for me to explain my symptoms using the definition of disability in the Equality Act, although I was not aware of this at the time.

There is increasing recognition of the impact endometriosis has on people with the condition in the workplace. The positive is that the responsibility to support women and menstruating people is on the employer, and there is now best practice guidance available to help employers to make these changes. People with disabilities are also protected under The Equality Act (2010). Endometriosis UK has a scheme in place for endometriosis-friendly employers, who sign up to the best practice guidelines for supporting people with endometriosis in the workplace. You can check if your employer is part of this scheme on the Endometriosis UK website.

Despite movement towards more recognition of endometriosis in the workplace, your ability to discuss your experience at work may still depend on the environment you work in and how able you feel to disclose. I had some experiences of discussing my symptoms at work which I felt were ignored and made me feel embarrassed for trying to discuss it. I also had more positive experiences which were met with compassion from others. When I made the decision to have a hysterectomy, I decided to be honest with my managers about my difficulties at work. This meant talking to a male manager about my endometriosis. I found this difficult because I had worked with him for years and told him very little about my physical health difficulties. This made the threat of disclosing now feel bigger, as I was worried he would not believe me based on his experience of me to that point. I rehearsed what I was going to say, and I was nervous about bringing this up. When I did have this conversation about my endometriosis it was met with compassion, and I was supported to take time off work for my surgery and recovery. My manager listened to me and what I needed, and I think it helped me to have a structure and a plan for that conversation, a skill we will look at later in this chapter. However, I still worry about missing work if I am unwell or in pain. I am also aware that despite the condition being incurable, I haven't revisited the impact of it with my manager much since returning from surgery. However, it now feels like that conversation will be easier because there is an awareness of my diagnosis and journey. Later in this chapter, we will look at some skills to help think about disclosure to others and what it is like to receive compassion from others. In chapter 8, we will look at bringing compassion to self in the absence of compassion from others.

Endometriosis and Friendships

I really value connection with other people in my life, and at times I feel that endometriosis has got in the way of this. I found it difficult to make new friends because I often needed to change social plans (or cancel them) in response to illness and flare ups. I didn't feel comfortable telling people that I had difficulties with my periods when we hadn't spent much time together and I found being unwell got in the way of spending time with new people. I might start new activities hoping to meet new people but would often end up discontinuing them in response to a change in my illness. I also didn't have a formal diagnosis until my 30s so I didn't really know what to tell people about what was happening to me.

Many of my friends have been in my life for decades. These friends have been aware of the progression of the illness as I have lived it. There were parts of the journey that facilitated disclosure, such as hospital admissions and surgeries, which meant my friends became aware that I was suffering, and this enabled me to talk to them more easily about why I had been in hospital and my health afterwards. However, I still did not disclose the extent of my experience as the threat of social disconnection loomed over all my relationships for a long time.

For me, the threat of losing my friendships or being perceived as weak by my friends got in the way of my life and at times my enjoyment of social events. There are many times when I have pushed through severe, persistent pain and illness rather than tell my friends how really I was feeling or cancel our plans. This means that some of our shared experiences carry very different memories for us – for example, my closest friends took me for a wonderful birthday meal one year. It was a high-end restaurant, booked a long time in advance. I was in a significant amount of pain that day, but rather than tell them this, I went ahead with the meal because I knew cancelling would incur a cost and I thought their enjoyment would be less if they were worried about me. I remember feeling like I was going to pass out walking to the restaurant and this impacted my enjoyment of the event. I have since talked about this with my friends and they were saddened and shocked that this meal, a happy memory for them, was so difficult for me. I realised that not only had I found the experience challenging and less enjoyable myself, but my friends also felt unhappy that we had not shared the experience in the way they had hoped. This was a trap I fell into many times, where I felt that sharing any part of my experience was not safe, so I shared none. My self-critic was in control telling me I would ruin the day if I told them how I was feeling. However, if I could have connected with some self-compassion, I might have been able to reassure myself that my friends would not see this as me ruining the day and this might have helped me to navigate that experience differently. It may also have allowed me to connect with the compassion my friends could have offered (other-to-self).

It may be that you are also finding times when you disconnect from your friends, or you push yourself to connect with others in ways that are unhelpful for you. I would encourage you to think about how you can begin to be open with others around you in a way that promotes and maintains connection. CFT is all about finding balance. We can think about how to move towards balance by sharing the experience with others and utilising the support that is available to us which may then allow us to maintain the relationships that are important. In chapter 9, we will think about examples of this when we learn about compassionate behaviour.

Endometriosis and Romantic Relationships

Endometriosis UK highlights that endometriosis can impact working lives, childcare, everyday tasks, and social lives which can place a couple under strain in a variety of ways including financial, emotional, and psychological pressure. In addition, the difficulties we have highlighted in this book in terms of access to treatment and healthcare appointments can be frustrating and difficult for both partners. Research indicates that endometriosis can place significant strain on relationships because of social withdrawal, painful sex, and challenges for partners in tolerating the constancy of the disease (Brown, 2007; Butt and Chesla, 2007; Hudson et al., 2016). Research also highlights the impact of endometriosis on both couples' mental health (Schick et al., 2022).

The impact of endometriosis on your romantic relationships might be different depending on when your symptoms start and where your relationship is at that time. I had suffered with symptoms of endometriosis throughout my life, so all my long-term romantic partners were aware this was a problem for me. The extent of their awareness differed depending on the impact the condition was having on me at the time and my own understanding of what was happening. This meant the conversation about the problems with my periods was an early part of any new relationship.

Although I was aware that there was 'a problem' with my periods for a long time, I did not understand the impact that was going to have on me as the condition progressed. I met my husband when I was 21 years old – at that time, I had worries about my fertility, recurrent UTIs, some discomfort during sexual intercourse, back pain, migraines, leg pain, left sided pain, and fatigue. I also had good days. I had no idea how my symptoms would change in the years after that. At that time, I was not even fully aware that they could. As time went on, my symptoms did change. I had multiple hospital admissions, surgery, worsening of existing symptoms, new symptoms including significant pain during intercourse, and I became increasingly disabled by my illness.

This made me feel guilty that I was no longer able to do the things I had done at the start of our relationship. At times, I felt like I wasn't even the same person. Endometriosis UK highlights how a couple's relationship can involve elements of care from one person to the other. Although I continue to find it difficult to accept, my husband took on a caring role at times in our relationship and marriage. He did most of the housework and many household tasks that were difficult for me. This dynamic became something that neither of us was fully aware of until after my surgery. For example, if we went out for coffee and there was a queue, he would always stand in the queue, and I would sit down. If something heavy needed lifting, he would lift it. It helped me to not have to ask him to do these things or for support in this way, but I still felt guilt and sadness about it at times. This was particularly evident when he needed support too, whether because he was also tired or unwell in some way, but I could not always provide that for him. For us, endometriosis was like a third wheel in our relationship – it was external to us as a couple but interfered with our dynamic and daily life. It is not something you can get rid of, it is always there and present and can make it harder to find a balance between the two of you.

When I used online support groups, I would often read about the experiences of other people who had not been supported in the way I have been by partners and family members. The phrase 'this is not what they signed up for' seemed to be a common feature of conversation when talking about romantic relationships. Many people (me included) worried about being a burden to their partners or families or holding them back from important experiences. This made me think of the activation of threat in these relationships – the idea that we were a burden to our partners, friends, or families and that could mean they would reject or abandon us. There was a sense that partners were giving up something by being with someone with endometriosis – perhaps the option to be with someone 'normal'. For some people I have met, their relationships had ended, and this had sometimes been connected with the impact endometriosis had on the couple. Personally, I often felt guilty about the impact my illness had on my husband and later, on our life as a family. At times, this pushed me towards a 'please response' to manage that threat, where I would try to go along with what I felt he or my family needed to make them happy but often at a high cost to myself. However, when it is estimated that one in ten women suffer with endometriosis, I think we need to recognise that we are not undeserving of love because of our condition and difficulties.

Endometriosis UK highlights that partners can often be a key source of support for a person living with endometriosis, which was my experience. It may be that relationships need to change to navigate the impact of the disease, but it does not mean that people with endometriosis cannot have meaningful, loving, and satisfying relationships. However, if you are in a relationship where you feel unsafe or at risk, you can access support for domestic violence and abuse. I have included information on these organisations in the additional support section at the end of this book.

Sex and Intimacy

I am not an expert in sexual therapy and although I want to acknowledge the impact of endometriosis on sex and intimacy, I am not going to discuss sexual intercourse in any detail within this chapter. It is essential to acknowledge that most of the research in this area focusses on heterosexual couples, and we are still expanding the evidence base for same-sex couples and for the LGBTQ+ community. As a heterosexual, cisgender woman, I also cannot personally speak to the challenges that are faced by members of the LGBTQ+ community. I hope that the information contained in this chapter can be utilised by all people living with endometriosis, although I recognise that there may be additional considerations for members of the LGBTQ+ community including the possibility that both partners may have endometriosis.

If you are finding it difficult to manage the impact of endometriosis on your sex life, you may want to access specialist support such as sexual therapy or couples counselling, which can be helpful to support couples to navigate their sexual relationship. Information on accessing further support is included in the resources section of this book. You can also find guidance on sex from Endometriosis UK.

Some of the physical symptoms associated with endometriosis can impact sex and physical intimacy for couples. This might include pain during sexual intercourse (dyspareunia), bleeding during or after sex, reduced sexual desire, pain, and/or discomfort associated with orgasm.

There are other factors that can also impact sex and physical intimacy including low mood, low self-esteem, body shame, medication, and fertility difficulties. All these experiences can activate our threat system and our self-critic. When sex becomes associated with pain, it can become an activity that activates our threat system. We might face a double threat of both pain and self-criticism which might lead to us feeling disconnected from our partners.

When sex becomes something that activates threat, it can also become something that both partners may want to avoid. The person with endometriosis may want to avoid experiencing the pain, and a partner without endometriosis may avoid sex or physical intimacy as they do not want to cause their partner any pain or suffering. It can be difficult to communicate this with each other and to find ways other of maintaining connection. Endometriosis UK highlights the importance of finding intimacy in other ways as well as maintaining clear communication with your partner. This is important because physical intimacy can be very difficult at times. For me, it wasn't only sexual intimacy that was impacted. During a flare up, I didn't want to be touched at all. I needed to be alone, with hot water bottles and pain relief to try to navigate the acute pain and distress that I experienced during this time. This meant that other forms of physical intimacy, such as cuddling on the sofa, or connecting emotionally by talking through what was happening, weren't always possible either. Being able to communicate what was happening at these times, usually after the acute phased had passed, helped me and my husband to understand that this was not about rejection of each other – it was about survival in that moment and that when that moment passed, we would come back to each other to recover, reconnect, and rebuild. However, it took time to have those conversations and build that understanding. At times, endometriosis could get in the way and make us feel disconnected from each other, so we needed to find ways to navigate that. In some couples, the challenges posed by endometriosis in a relationship can result in a cycle of both partners feeling distant from each other, as neither feels able to connect with the other. Sometimes this might lead to other difficulties such as feeling rejected or unloved by the other.

Throughout this book, we have focused on how the activation of our threat system can inhibit us from communication with others and other safety strategies that might have unintended consequences. Physical intimacy is one area where threat can be activated, so we are focusing on being able to connect with each other in different ways. We know that communicating effectively within a relationship is essential to maintain supportive, secure bonds with our partner. In this chapter, we will look at applying the skills of compassion to our intimate relationships and improving communication with our partners as a way of maintaining connection and intimacy. We will also think about communicating our needs in other relationships in our lives.

Talking about Endometriosis with Others: The Search for Support

As discussed at the beginning of this chapter, I had many experiences of reaching out to others for support that were not positive. Although these experiences were all different, they were also similar in that they all left me feeling misunderstood by other people. This activated my threat system and my old brain patterns of anxiety and avoidance. Sometimes I would experience the responses of other people as shaming (see chapter 6). This happened most often in moments of small disclosure, for example, declining a long walk after a pub lunch due to pain which was met with a response of 'it's only a walk, we won't be more than an hour'. I realise that I was trying to assert my needs, but the people I was speaking to were missing the wider context, and this led to 'shoulds' being applied to me sometimes by others (external) and sometimes by myself (internal). Talking about your endometriosis is a personal decision. It might take a long time, and you might choose to share different things in different relationships. However, taking some control of your narrative and being able to share this experience with others may mean you can share your distress and be met with care, compassion, and support from others, even if this is not everyone.

When I began to talk about my endometriosis, I learnt that it was helpful to focus on what I needed to communicate so the message was understood. This may also be helpful for you. In my walk example, I would often say something like 'no thanks, I think I will stay here' which meant people did not understand I was in pain and did not feel able to go and would therefore try to encourage me to join, activating my threat. I also didn't want to share everything about my endometriosis or experience in that situation. It is focussing on the part you need people to understand at that moment, so you feel more empowered about your decisions and other people can better understand your needs. In this example, to someone I did not know well, I could have said 'I don't want to join the walk today. I am going to go home, but I hope you all have a great time and I will catch up with you afterwards.' For someone close to me, I could say 'I am on my period suffering with my endo, I can't walk today can we please go home?'.

Being able to talk about your endometriosis, your symptoms, and your experiences is unlikely to ever mean sharing everything with everyone. This is about sharing what you need to and making an informed choice, rather than falling into unhelpful patterns.

You may be able to find practical solutions to maintaining connection with other people and utilising the support they can offer you. Having conversations with others and beginning to think about endometriosis as something that needs to be managed rather than cured might be helpful in beginning to consider practical solutions that will help you maintain connection. Practical solutions might include:

- Trying to find a balance between time alone and time together.
- Finding other ways to promote physical intimacy such as touching, cuddling, kissing, holding hands. If this isn't possible, working on communicating with the other person what you are experiencing, so you maintain connection with them in other ways.
- Accepting offers of support from others that make daily life easier (e.g. support with household tasks).

Receiving Compassion from Others

My hope is that as you begin to talk to other people about your experience, you will begin to receive compassion and support (other-self flow of compassion). My experience of sharing my experience more openly is that I have received more compassion from others than I have expected, which has been difficult to receive at times. As we have learnt, there are barriers to connecting with compassion. Compassion requires us to turn towards suffering and to have the knowledge, wisdom, and motivation to want to alleviate it. I think this is helpful to apply to our decision making about sharing our experiences with others – we need to be able to share both our experience and also what we need from the other person to support us. Many of the challenges of endometriosis cannot be solved or fixed, so we may just need company, acknowledgement, or space. Communicating this can enable us to receive the care and connection that we need from others. It can also make them feel more empowered in how to support us. My husband often wanted to 'know what to do' so he could make me feel better or make the problem go away – when we hadn't communicated well, I would become annoyed by this because there wasn't anything he could do, and it wasn't going to go away. However, I recognise that he was trying to help and give support – but the support I needed was an acknowledgement that this was hard, and he was there for me.

In chapter 4, we talked about some of the barriers to compassion. We know that connecting with the flows of compassion can be difficult for a variety of reasons and receiving compassion requires us to open up and be vulnerable. This can be very threatening, particularly if you have learnt that opening up to others is met with rejection or negativity. For me, compassionate or empathetic responses from other people could trigger off thoughts of that person seeing me as weak, and this would pull me back towards dismissing or minimising my experience. Sometimes receiving compassion might also activate thoughts and feelings associated with being a burden to others.

It can help to spend time opening your mind to receiving compassion from others as research has shown that the experience of being and feeling cared for can help us to manage our distress (Irons and Beaumont, 2017), which might make us feel more able to manage the challenges we are facing in our life and be more able to connect with others and the world around us. This is because it activates our soothing systems, which helps to calms the threat system. Connection, compassion, and empathy are the antidotes to threat.

One way to begin to connect with the care and kindness of others is to be able to connect with this in our daily life. As we know, when we are in threat, it is difficult to notice moments of compassion from other people. For example, if I had been at work all day, was in significant pain, bleeding, fatigued and nauseous, I did not notice the person who held the door for me as I left the office. When I got home and my husband made dinner for us, I felt guilt rather than care and connection. We can use our compassionate self (chapter 7) to self-correct and bring compassion to ourselves, letting us know that it is understandable we are struggling today and we need support to care for ourselves in this moment. We can also begin to use our skills to allow us to connect with the compassion offered to us by others and accepting this, which may reduce our distress as we connect with multiple flows of compassion in one moment (self-self, other-self, in this example).

You can use the exercise below to begin to explore connecting with compassion from others by thinking about how to share your experience and your needs with them.

There is a worksheet below to help you think through the decision to talk to someone about your symptoms and experience and what you might want to say. We can never predict exactly how another person will respond to us sharing our experience, but if we think carefully about who and what to share, hopefully we can access people who are able to offer compassion.

Am I comfortable with this person? Do I feel they could offer me support and compassion?	
Do I feel able to speak about my illness? Do I feel able to explain this to another person? If so, how would I do this?	
Is there something I need support with now? Could I ask for this support in relation to that problem?	
Can I create space and time for this conversation? How would I do this?	
What will help me to manage my own emotional response to this conversation? How can I take care of myself at this time?	

You might do this next part of the exercise now, or when you have sought support from another person. It is likely that you will repeat this exercise more than once as you explore connecting with others in different ways and in different relationships. Not all these experiences may be positive or go the way you are expecting, but this is a process of trial and error, as you work out what works for you and the relationships that are important in your life. If this exercise is challenging, revisit chapter 6 to bring compassion to the challenge and remind yourself of the motivation behind this work – to connect with your suffering and to do something about it.

What was it like to use support from another person? Did you feel there were things that you gained from this? What would help you to do this again in the future?

_____
_____
_____
_____
_____

Developing a Compassionate Other

You may not have anyone in your life that you feel able to talk to about your endometriosis. Many people do not have access to the support that I was fortunate to receive from people around me and the compassionate healthcare professionals who helped to change my life. Even if you do have people in your life who support you, there may still be times that you don't feel able to connect with them (I frequently experienced this). It can therefore be helpful to develop a compassionate other – this is an image of someone or something that is there to bring compassion, kindness, wisdom, and strength to us at times of challenge. Imagery is often used in CFT as it can be powerful in helping us to connect with feelings of calm, safety, and soothing. Using an exercise like this might make you feel what you might feel if it was a real person responding to you in this way. Remember we are not trying to replace real people with a compassionate other, but this exercise might help you move towards accepting compassion from people in your life if this is something that is difficult. It can also allow you to connect with compassion from others at times this might be difficult or unavailable in our lives.

Sometimes people find it difficult to develop a clear image of a compassionate other or might feel uncomfortable thinking about another person having compassion for them. Don't worry if this is the case. The aim is to focus on a compassionate other wanting to be here for you and support you, even if they are not clear in your mind. If this still feels challenging, you might want to revisit barriers to compassion in chapter 4. This exercise is adapted from the resources online at the Compassionate Mind Foundation. Remember to complete this exercise in a position which is comfortable for you.

Take a moment to engage your soothing rhythm breathing.

When you are ready, pay attention to your posture and facial expression. See if you want to soften this or let go of any tension in your body as you prepare to connect with your compassionate other.

Take a moment to think about someone who has been compassionate to you in the past. This person could be real, or they could be fictional. Your compassionate other can also be a mash up of characteristics that you experience as compassionate and nothing like a person you've ever seen, met, or imagined before. You can take pieces of all the people who come to mind. Take a moment to think about this person, or people, and the qualities of compassion they have.

Bring to mind how this person or people look and what they sound like. How do you know this person is committed to supporting you?

Now think about what you need to connect with the compassion this person is offering you. It might be scary to connect with this, particularly if it is unfamiliar to you. Remember that this is understandable and just take a moment to sit with knowing that this person is with you in this experience.

Take a few moments to sit with these thoughts and questions in your mind. When you are ready, turn your attention back to your breathing, slowly open your eyes, and connect with the world around you.

After you have completed this exercise, use the space below to describe or draw your compassionate other. Try bringing your compassionate other to mind at times of challenge and see how this feels for you. Continue to practice bringing this person to mind and connecting with the compassionate and caring commitment they offer you.

_____
_____
_____
_____
_____

Once you have developed a compassionate other, or begun to explore connecting with other people in your life, you may begin to feel more able to speak about your experiences and access support from those around you. However, living with endometriosis means being able to access support both in your own relationships and in terms of accessing healthcare. I found that this required me to be assertive at times, something I found almost impossible if I was stuck in a tricky loop or overwhelmed by threat. In the final part of this chapter we will think about how to bring together the skills learnt so far to help us be assertive in our relationships with others and how we can use these skills when accessing healthcare services and making treatment decisions.

Being Assertive

I found it difficult to assert myself in many situations related to my endometriosis. Many of my personal examples relate to accessing healthcare, as this was a challenge for me. Research from the All Parlimentary Group on Endometriosis (2020) shows I am not alone in this experience. Prior to getting a diagnosis, 58% of women accessed their GP more than 10 times, 43% visited doctors in hospital more than 5 times and 53% visited A&E. However, you may not experience this as there are many healthcare professionals who are committed to supporting people with endometriosis. Recently in my GP surgery, I found a variety of leaflets about endometriosis which had not been there previously, highlighting to me how much things are changing. The examples that come to mind from my past experience are booking appointments with the GP with the 'same problem' that I had been told had no solution previously and asserting myself if a course of treatment wasn't working. This was particularly the case with hormonal treatments as I was often told they need time to 'settle'. I persevered with at least two hormonal treatments, each for over 12 months, because I was encouraged to by the GP, and it took me a long time to be able to assert myself and say this was not working for me, and I wanted an alternative. Being assertive is an area in which we can also use our compassionate mind to help us.

As you will know by this point in the book, the first step to making a change is naming where we are experiencing this difficulty. Let's start by thinking about situations where you find it difficult to be assertive. I have given examples from my own experience on the left. Underneath, you may want to revisit your four-part formulation from chapter 3, to think about why it is understandable that it might be difficult for you to be assertive in these situations and what your fears are of behaving assertively. In the final part of the worksheet, we are bringing together our difficulties with the wisdom and strength of our compassionate self.

Difficulties in being assertive	
My examples	Your examples
Booking GP Appointments	
Talking to the GP	
Asking for a different approach to treatment	
Saying no to people when the request would impact my health	
Not expressing my needs or preferences to others	
Asking for different/more support at work	

(*Continued*)

(*Continued*)

What underlies these difficulties.	
Repeated, difficult experiences with GPs Difficult response from other people Internalised view of myself as the problem, weak, unable to cope Lack of trust in my own judgement/assessment of my own needs	
Fears of being assertive	
Fear that if I started to say what I wanted or needed, I would be perceived as aggressive, over-reacting, or mentally unwell.	
Bringing compassion to being assertive	
My compassionate other knows that it is difficult for me to be assertive because of my past experiences and the beliefs I have held about myself, which are untrue. It is understandable that this is difficult for me, given the experiences I have had. My compassionate other wants to support me with this difficulty and help me to move forward.	

When you feel able to move towards being more assertive, remember our theme on naming – this time we are 'Naming that need'. You might find this framework helpful to do this.

I need ... Because ... I need you to ... so that ...

An example might be, 'I need to change the treatment I am on because this is not working for me. I need you to talk me through the other treatment options available so we can find a treatment that is more effective at managing my symptoms.'

You may want to use this exercise to prepare for appointments or difficult conversations. It can also help to have conversations with partners and loved ones. I found that going through what I needed to say prior to appointments or difficult conversations was helpful for me in making myself clear at a time when threat was active for me and it was harder to keep my systems in balance.

In chapter 9, we are going to look at bringing our skills to some of the symptoms associated with endometriosis as we continue to work on balancing our three systems at times of challenge.

Summary

- Endometriosis can impact our relationships with others as well as our relationship with ourselves. Different relationships will be impacted differently by the condition, and it can be helpful to think about how to manage the impact endometriosis has in different relationships.
- At work and in friendships, it might be helpful to think about how and when to disclose your endometriosis and the impact it has on you so you can access support available.
- The impact of endometriosis can be significant in romantic relationships. It can impact the communication and connection with your romantic partner as well as sex and physical intimacy.
- We can connect with our compassionate self to help us make decisions about how to talk about our endometriosis with others. It will not always be possible, or appropriate to share our experience, but we are aiming to make a choice that may allow us to receive compassion from others who are able to give it. Receiving compassion can be difficult, and we may need to practice this.
- We can develop a compassionate other to help us to practice receiving compassion from another person. This can be in

addition to our compassionate selves as these different exercises allow us to connect with different flows of compassion.
- Being able to share our experiences with others sometimes requires us to be assertive, and we can bring compassion to this challenge. This aims to help us clearly communicate our needs so we are more likely to receive a compassionate response from others, connecting us with the flow of other-to-self.

9 Relationship with Endometriosis

Introduction

In chapters 7 and 8, we have talked about the impact that endometriosis can have on our relationship with ourselves and with other people. In this chapter, we will think about the relationship we have with some of the symptoms and difficulties associated with the condition, in other words, our relationship with endometriosis. As we discussed in chapter 2, there are many symptoms that can be associated with endometriosis, and it is not possible to consider all of them here. Instead, I have focussed on the symptoms that caused me the most distress and were the most frequent. I am not going to consider the medical interventions available for these symptoms as there is information available from other resources (see references) about the treatments for endometriosis, and these are summarised earlier in this book. In this chapter we will think about how to bring our compassionate mind to some of these symptoms to reduce the distress associated with them. Connecting with compassion to help manage the symptoms of the condition and their impact will not make them go away. However, I found it did enable me to cope at times of struggle. Although it is not possible to cover every symptom and difficulty associated with endometriosis here, my hope is that you can take these examples and then apply the skills to other areas of your experience.

Endometriosis and Fertility

Not everyone will want to have children in their lifetime, so this may not apply to you in which case, you may choose to skip this section. However, fertility is a concern for many people living with endometriosis and one that I felt could not be overlooked in this book. You may think about fertility at several points in your journey, perhaps you are not currently considering your fertility, or it may be a significant part of your life right now. I was aware of possible difficulties with my fertility due to my 'problem periods' from when I was 16 years old and a GP told me I probably wouldn't be able to have a baby, something I was not considering at the time. This information was inaccurate as research from Endometriosis UK suggests that 60–70% of people living with endometriosis conceive without medical intervention. However, it stuck in my mind, and I believed that I might not be able to conceive. Like many people, I continued to be given mixed messages about the possible impact of my difficulties on my fertility. Although not all people have fertility difficulties, one in seven heterosexual couples in the UK do. For those women and birthing people who do have fertility difficulties, the prevalence of endometriosis can be as high as 30–50% (Endometriosis UK, 2023a; Meuleman, 2009). I was also told by a GP that pregnancy would cure my endometriosis, advice which is untrue (BBC News, 2021). For some women and birthing people, symptoms improve during pregnancy but can return after birth once periods start again. For me, although some of my difficulties were different during pregnancy, the pain was persistent and more severe. I also had bleeding during pregnancy and some of my bladder and bowel symptoms continued.

All these messages contributed to the activation of my threat system in relation to my fertility. As we learnt earlier in this book, our threat system can be activated by both the imagined fear of something and the reality. For me, my threat system was activated by the uncertainty of whether I would have difficulties with my fertility once I tried to conceive even though the reality turned out to be different. You may want to pause here to think about what threats are present for you in relation to your fertility. Later in this section, we will think about bringing compassion to the difficult emotions that might be present in relation to these threats.

Examples from my experience	Examples from your experience
Uncertainty about my fertility. High anxiety about stopping contraceptives to try to conceive and the impact this would have on my symptoms. High anxiety whilst trying to conceive. Worries about losing my baby when I became pregnant.	

For me, the reality of trying to conceive was straightforward. I was able to conceive without medical intervention or assistance, and this was not a long journey. However, my decisions relating to my fertility and my experience of having a baby were influenced by the fear I had about not being able to conceive which had activated my threat system. As a result, I felt that I needed to prioritise having a baby earlier in my life than I would have done if I did not have endometriosis. For other people, concerns about their fertility may mean they decide not to have children, or they delay trying to conceive because of the impact endometriosis has on their lives (Endometriosis UK, 2023a).

I think it is essential to recognise when we talk about fertility, we are not only talking about the ability to have a baby. I was apprehensive writing this section, as my self-critic shouted, 'you had a baby, what do you know about fertility?'. However, my fertility was something that I considered multiple times in my journey. Prior to having my daughter, I had imagined a life with more than one child. However, I had a difficult pregnancy and challenging birth experience. I had early bleeding which increased my fear of miscarriage, significant nausea throughout my pregnancy, pelvic pain which was debilitating, and severe migraines. I was suspected of pre-term labour resulting in hospital admissions and bed rest for most of the third trimester. I was induced and this was a painful experience where I felt out of control. I believed I would cope well with the pain of labour as I was used to severe pain, but I did not cope the way I thought I would. This activated my threat system and initially I was very critical of myself and my birth – thinking I should have coped better and been more in control of myself and my emotions. After my delivery, I used many of the skills we have learnt in this book to connect with self-to-self compassion about my birth experience which helped me to approach this experience differently.

After my daughter was born, my endometriosis seemed to worsen significantly. I had multiple ovarian cysts that ruptured, increasing pelvic pain which restricted my daily life, increased bleeding which was more irregular, anaemia, and fatigue. After I had my daughter, I opted to try the Mirena coil (a small t-shaped frame which has the hormone progesterone on it and is inserted into the womb), but this did not control my symptoms, and they seemed to worsen. I had this removed but spent around 12 months feeling increasingly unwell which was attributed to being a new mum, feeling tired with a new baby, and ongoing symptoms. I was so used to having some pain, discomfort, and fatigue that when the GP told me there was no problem, I returned to my usual assumptions, that I was coping badly with normal problems, and I continued to struggle. When my daughter was 18 months old, I collapsed at home. I was rushed into hospital and initially treated for a kidney infection before being discharged. I asked for a gynaecology referral at this time, but this did not happen as the doctors felt it wasn't warranted, and I wanted to go home to my baby daughter, so I didn't insist. I then collapsed again, with early indicators for sepsis (my second episode) and I was taken back to hospital in an ambulance. It was discovered that I had a severe pelvic infection, and this had caused damage to my fallopian tubes resulting in surgery and a stay in hospital. The surgeon told me it was likely this infection had been there and spreading for around 12 months, which in my view explains my year of illness. The damage to my fallopian tubes placed me at high risk of ectopic pregnancy and I was advised I may have difficulties conceiving. If I did conceive, I would need early scans in any future pregnancies to ensure they were not ectopic which can be life threatening. My difficult pregnancy, birth, and then subsequent increased risk of ectopic pregnancies all contributed to further threat activation in relation to my fertility.

The worsening of my symptoms became increasingly debilitating, and this impacted my role as a mum. I couldn't run around the garden, stand watching in the park, sit on the floor to play with toys, or pick my daughter up as she got bigger. I felt like I couldn't be there for the child I had in the way I wanted to be, and the idea of another pregnancy scared me. My husband and I also felt that our family was complete as a three and although this was different to our previous expectations, it felt like something we were able to accept. As I discussed treatment options available to me with my final two consultants hysterectomy became one I felt I needed to consider. Some people, like me, might opt for radical surgery as part of their treatment. This is a significant decision in relation to fertility as it will mean being unable to carry a baby. In addition, hysterectomy is not a cure for endometriosis. Although it will stop your periods, you may continue to have other symptoms associated with the disease. This was a point of dilemma for me as I was giving up the option to have more children without knowing whether the surgery would help with the difficulties I had. Although I knew that hysterectomy would relieve some of the symptoms I had due to adenomyosis, I didn't know which of my symptoms related to which diagnosis. I spent several months working through this decision in therapy and with the support of my family.

When I reflect on this journey, what I remember most is the many difficult emotions I felt during this experience. Each step felt that it brought up difficult emotions and it is these emotions that I felt compassion helped me to manage.

Fertility and Managing Difficult Emotions

When I sat to write this part of the book, I found it difficult to think about what aspect of my fertility journey was the most challenging and the skills I used to manage it. I thought about the first conversations with my husband fearing that he might not want to be with me if I couldn't have a baby, stopping the contraceptive pill to allow my periods to return for the first time in over a decade, then waiting to see if I was pregnant and finally letting go of my fertility completely at 33 years old. As I thought about it, I remembered all the emotions connected with this part of my journey and it is still difficult. I realised that it was the difficult emotions I experienced throughout this time that I was able to bring compassion to and this is what helped me to cope. I couldn't change the experiences I was having, or the emotions I felt and sometimes still feel, but I could manage those emotions in a way that allowed me to process them safely, without feeling out of control which was how I felt in so many other areas of my experience. CFT reminds us that all emotions have a function – it was not my fault that my fertility decisions were complex or that I had faced challenges during my pregnancy. My emotions had reminded me that this was a difficult time and experience for me. It was (and still is) ok that I feel sad about my experience and the impact it had on my life and our family. It is also ok that I chose, with the support of my husband, not to have more children, in part because of the impact it could have on me physically and psychologically. I have to regularly remind myself of this compassionate decision making, as I still get asked by all kinds of people whether I considered having more children or why I have 'just one' child as if it is something to be ashamed of.

Everyone will feel differently about their fertility and the threats associated with this. It is recognised that difficulties with fertility can lead to feelings of anger, inadequacy, and failure (Endometriosis UK, 2023a). Stress, depression, and anxiety are also common experiences for those struggling with fertility (Doyle and Carballedo, 2014). We can use compassion to help us to tolerate difficult emotions that may come up for us in our endometriosis and fertility journey. Sometimes it can be scary to connect with what we are feeling, as we can worry that if we allow ourselves to feel the difficult emotion it might overwhelm us. This reminds me of something people sometimes say when they access therapy 'if I start crying, or thinking about this, then I will never be able to stop'. Although it may feel this way, we know this is untrue – difficult emotions will pass, and being able to connect with them with compassion can support us with allowing this process to happen. The exercise below (adapted from Irons and Beaumont, 2017) is designed to bring our compassionate mind and self to our difficult feelings which may come up at any point in our journey, perhaps in relation to our fertility or other challenges associated with endometriosis. As with all the exercises in this book, find a position which is comfortable for you and start with your soothing rhythm breathing.

> *Take a few moments to connect with your breathing and when you are ready, engage a soothing rhythm to your breath. Focus on this for a few moments.*
>
> *When you are ready, bring to mind your compassionate self. Remember the qualities of compassion they bring to you – they are motivated to help and support you, and they do this with wisdom and strength.*
>
> *Now think about the emotion that is difficult for you right now. You might remember the last time you felt this – what was it that made you feel this emotion?*
>
> *What would your compassionate self say or do to help you with this emotion? How might they help you with this feeling?*
>
> *Allow yourself to be with this difficult feeling, with the strength and support from your compassionate self. Notice what happens to this feeling with the courage and wisdom that your compassionate self gives you.*
>
> *When you are ready, spend a few moments refocussing on your soothing rhythm breathing before you open your eyes and reconnect with the present moment.*

I still feel the sadness, grief, and anger that endometriosis dictated my decisions about my fertility. However, I connect with the strength, kindness, and wisdom of my compassionate self that these were the right decisions for me, and this has allowed me to accept the challenges I faced. I recognise that having my daughter has helped me in this, because I do feel thankful to have had a baby as I know this will not be the case for everyone with endometriosis. However, whatever your journey, I hope that bringing compassion to your difficult emotions is helpful.

Endometriosis, Persistent Pain, and Disability

Pain is a normal part of being human and essential to our survival. Like other threats in our lives, it serves a survival function. Pain is a trigger for our internal alarm system (see chapter 5). If we can understand this pain as unthreatening, for example, a paper cut, then we are likely to be able to quickly turn down our alarm. We can sometimes control our response to pain in the face of more important goals, for example, some people will run a marathon through pain because it is important to them to cross the finish line. This may be both threat and drive systems working together to push forward or working with a dominant drive system to achieve the goal despite the threat system being active in response to the pain or discomfort.

Over 60% of people with endometriosis experience chronic pelvic pain, and people with endometriosis are 13 times more likely to report abdominal pain than those without endometriosis (Maddern et al., 2020). Pain can vary from person to person. Some people may experience pain that comes and goes in line with their menstrual cycle, and other people may experience persistent pain. The pain associated with endometriosis can be varied – I had severe cramping pains during my period (which after childbirth I realised felt like contractions); stabbing in my ovaries which could cause me to pass out; constant aching, shooting pains in my legs, heaviness and burning down my legs, back pain, pelvic pain, and many others.

There are factors that can influence how pain due to endometriosis is experienced. For example, the location and the depth of the lesions, as well as presence of any adhesions, can impact on how pain is felt. Abdominal pain can sometimes spread to the back, legs, and hips, and pain may be impacted by certain triggers such as sex or going to the toilet (NHS, 2022b).

Of all the symptoms I experienced, the most debilitating, distressing, and difficult to manage was pain. In the early stages of my journey, this pain was most acute around my period and would reduce when my bleeding had stopped. This meant that the first treatment I received was the combined pill which I took without a break, as not having a period meant I avoided the acute episodes of pain. However, as my endometriosis progressed the pain became more persistent. I cannot remember a day without pain from around the age of 21, until my hysterectomy and excision surgery at age 33. Persistent pain (sometimes called chronic or long-term pain) is pain that continues for three months or more and does not respond to usual medical treatment or continues despite treatment (The Pain Toolkit, 2023).

There are many treatment options available to help with pain in endometriosis. Endometriosis UK recommends heat, painkillers, physiotherapy, and TENS machines (an electrical device that uses electrical pulses to stimulate nerves and muscles to provide pain relief). In the UK, it is also possible to ask for a specialist referral to a pain clinic, although the availability of these will vary on where you live. I used all these methods at different times and some alternative therapies such as acupuncture to try to manage my pain. However, none of them completely controlled my pain, and I lived with persistent pain until my hysterectomy and excision surgery. Since my hysterectomy, I do experience some cyclical pain which I link to ovulation as I have one ovary left. However, this is a very different experience to the persistent pain I had before. As with other chapters in this book, I am not going to focus on the medical treatments available for pain as information on these is available elsewhere. Instead, I am going to focus on the psychological and emotional impact of persistent pain and how we can use compassion to manage the psychological impact of pain.

Persistent pain triggers the body's alarm system, but it does this repeatedly, often making it difficult to focus our attention on other things that are important in our lives. This is both distressing and depressing (Linton et al., 2011) as you are drawn away from things that activate drive and soothing and you become stuck in a cycle of threat. Your threat system draws so much of your attention, that it may be hard to even notice the other systems exist sometimes.

Pain was also one of the symptoms I found difficult to explain to other people, particularly people who had never experienced persistent pain (you can revisit chapter 8 to think about how you might communicate your experience of pain with others). On the occasions I did talk to others about how I was feeling, they would often say things like 'you just need to take a break', 'have a rest', or 'just be kind to yourself'. I found this very annoying, but it took me a long time to really understand why. It might seem obvious that if you are in pain or struggling, it might make sense to rest and recover. However, this is one of the difficulties living with persistent pain in endometriosis – unlike other pain episodes, rest does not necessarily lead to recovery. In my case, my self-critic would then show up, telling me that resting was pointless and would only confirm that I was useless and pathetic. If I rested when I was in pain, I thought I would end up doing this all the time and I would never achieve anything in my life. You can revisit the skills from previous chapters to think about how to bring your compassionate self to pain (chapter 7), how to reframe your internal narrative about pain (chapter 7), and how to communicate your pain with others (chapter 8).

One way to think about persistent pain from a compassion perspective is by using the model of persistent pain by Penlington et al., 2018 (see picture below). I have applied this cycle to the pain I experienced with endometriosis, and it may be a helpful way to understand the possible impact of your pain on your life and allow you to consider if there is anything you can change. We will go through this model in detail to help you think about how you might apply this to your own experience of pain. Later in this chapter, we will consider how you might utilise compassion to make those changes.

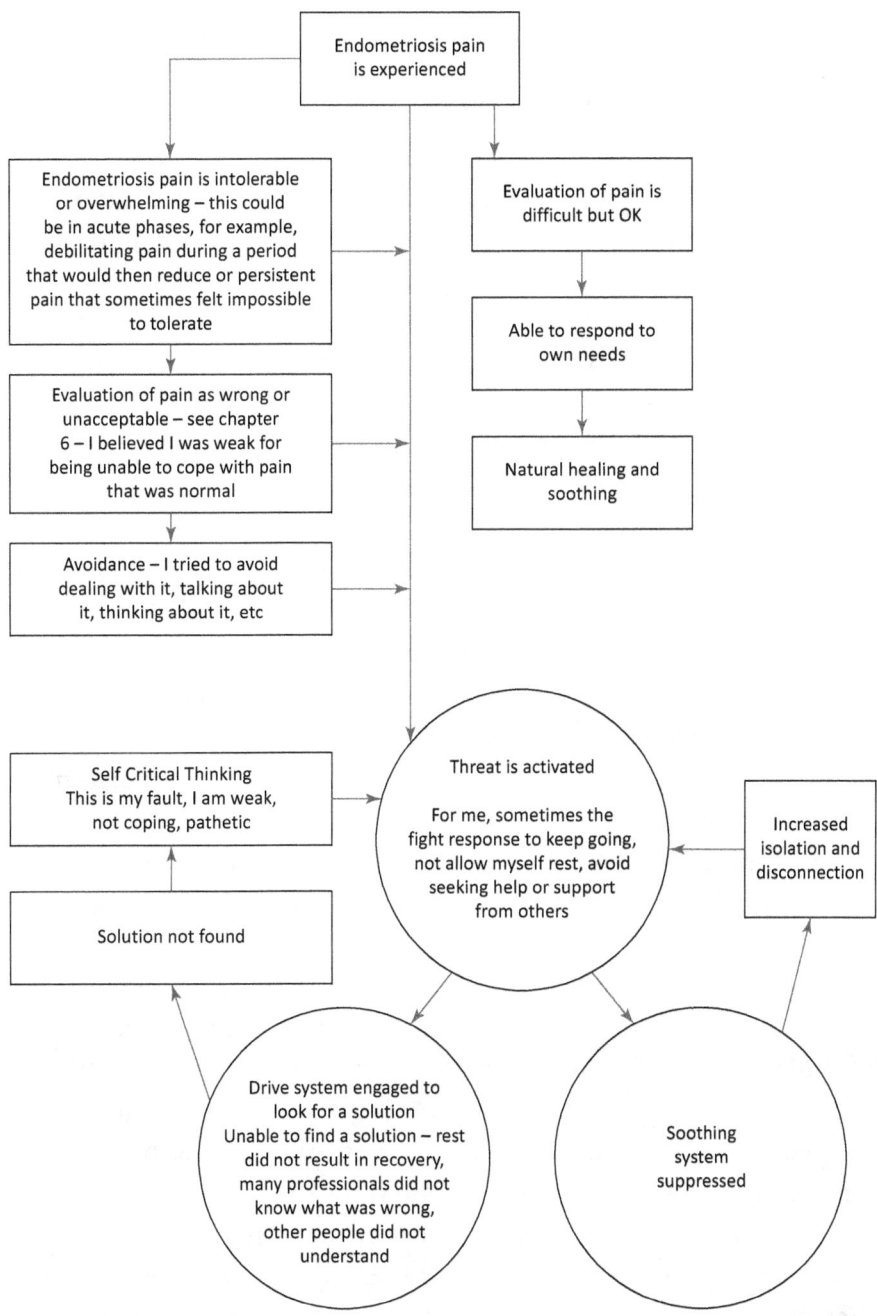

Three Systems Model of Persistent Pain: Adapted for this book from Penlington (2018) with permission from the author.

The impact of persistent pain on my life brings together many of the themes we have discussed in this book. The skills we have learnt can all be used to connect with compassion towards that experience. However, it is also the experience I found hardest to connect with across all three flows of compassion. I found it difficult to be compassionate to others when I was in pain and I was more irritable, which made me feel guilty. I found it difficult to connect with others, so their compassion was not available to me. I was fearful of connecting with compassion from others in relation to my pain as I believed they would see me as weak and unable to cope or possibly think I was lying. I didn't allow myself compassion because my self-critic and internal shame made me feel that I was not deserving of compassion because I was failing to manage a experience I believed was normal. This cycle kept me stuck in my distress and suffering both psychologically and physically.

For many people with endometriosis, me included, the pain and symptoms of endometriosis can be disabling, and it can be difficult to carry on with daily life. Prior to my hysterectomy, I reached a point in my journey where pushing on through pain driven by threat was becoming impossible. I was motivated to make changes for my family, as I wanted to be able to be present for my daughter and to show her that despite my challenges, I would be there for her. I could not do that if I had driven myself to the point of total collapse. All the skills we have discussed in this book can be used to connect with compassion for yourself and your experience at times of pain. Compassion does not mean you have to like or love what is happening, it means being able to approach what is happening with the qualities of compassion – strength, wisdom, kindness, and the motivation to alleviate the suffering. In endometriosis, motivation to change doesn't mean make it go away, it means being compassionate to the suffering you are experiencing in that moment. To this point, we have focussed on increasing our awareness and understanding of our experience and using psychological skills to manage this. I think pain requires us to also consider how we change our behaviour to be more compassionate towards ourselves. This is difficult, and for that reason, we will first consider what compassionate behaviour is and how this might look in endometriosis. We will then consider some of the challenges that come with making a change like this (and other changes discussed in this book) and how you might be able to approach doing something differently.

Compassionate Behaviour

Our behaviour, just like our thoughts and feelings, can be influenced by our threat system. When we are stuck in threat, we might behave differently and do things that might increase our suffering even if this is unintended (see chapter 3 to revisit the unintended consequences of safety behaviours). It is not our fault that we find ourselves behaving in ways that might not ultimately be helpful to us. However, compassionate behaviour means working on changing our behaviour to help us avoid patterns that might increase or maintain our distress, rather than reducing it.

Compassionate behaviour can easily be confused with doing something nice. Sometimes doing something nice is compassionate, but other times it might be a behaviour that is keeping us away from our distress. Imagine you have planned to go for a coffee with a close friend. The function of this coffee was to maintain social connection with this friend who is an important person in your life, someone you value and who you enjoy spending time with. When the day comes around, you have had some cramping and are feeling anxious about the possibility of bleeding whilst out at the cafe. Your threat system is activated, and you want to hide away from others, including your friend. You might think that self-compassion would mean cancelling the coffee and spending the morning in bed, watching your favourite TV shows. Although this might help you with managing the symptoms, it will take you away from the social connection with your friend that was the purpose of planning the coffee in the first place. Self-compassion might look like using the skills we have been learning in this book to do something that enables you to maintain that connection with your friend, despite the pain and discomfort you are feeling on that day. This is an example of being able to look towards the suffering, whilst also having the wisdom to do something about it. This might be explaining that you only want to go out for a short time, choosing somewhere you will feel more comfortable like meeting at home or opting for a video or telephone call instead. You might reschedule for another day and share with your friend how you are feeling. This allows you to maintain social connection, gain the support of your friend whilst also being compassionate to your own needs on that day.

Sometimes being compassionate to ourselves might involve giving ourselves the support we need to change patterns of behaviour that are not helping us. This doesn't mean that compassion doesn't sometimes look like spending the morning in bed, watching TV, or having a bubble bath. Self-compassion can look like all kind of things at different times, but it is important to remember that sometimes self-compassion looks like facing difficulties in our life differently.

Throughout this book, we have worked on identifying things we might avoid due to threat, and we have begun to develop skills to allow us to move away from avoidance and towards compassion. We have thought about how we can utilise compassion from others and compassion from ourselves to help us make these changes. Now let's look at some of the behavioural strategies that might further our journey towards self-compassion.

Using the Compassionate Self to Work with Difficulties

In this exercise, you might think about what is getting in the way of you making a change. For me, this was often the fear that things would get worse. I worried if I took time to rest, I wouldn't be able to get up again and keep going. I was worried if I told people about my difficulties, they would see me differently and as lesser. I feared I could go through a significant operation, lose my fertility, impact my family and life to then be more disabled than I was already. It can help to spend some time bringing your attention to these worries that make you feel stuck before you begin to attempt making a change.

> *As always, find a comfortable position and use your soothing rhythm breathing to bring to mind your compassionate self. Spend a few moments connecting with this part of you, so you can draw on its wisdom and strength.*
>
> *Now use this part of you to think about what is stopping you from facing your fears or making a change in your life now? Is there something getting in the way of changing? If there is, what would it be like to let go of this and take a first step towards the change? How might you do this? Why is it important for you to make this change? What impact will it have on your life if you are able to do this?*
>
> *Spend a few moments thinking over these questions. When you are ready, focus back on your breath before opening your eyes and connecting with the world around you.*

You may want to make some notes after this exercise, so you can bring these ideas and reflections to the final part of this chapter.

_____
_____
_____
_____
_____

Making Changes

Throughout this book, we have used imagery as a way of understanding our self-criticism and developing our compassionate other and compassionate self. We can use the same techniques to imagine facing our fears before we try it in real life. I found this very helpful because the outcome of making a change is always uncertain and using imagery helped me to find ways of managing that uncertainty and begin to believe I could cope with that challenging situation.

There may be specific situations which you would like to deal with differently in your life. Some of these might feel bigger or scarier than others, or they may all feel different at different times. Start with making a list of the situations which you find difficult and would like to change. Once you have thought of some changes, think about which ones feel achievable right now, and which ones feel more difficult or possibly even unimaginable. Reorder your list from 'I think I could work on this right now' to 'I need more time to get here'. I would suggest you then start from right now and work towards the things that feel more challenging. This is because if you start with things that feel more achievable right now, you are more likely to achieve them, and this will then increase your confidence and motivation to work towards the things that are more difficult. However, you can approach this in whatever way feels right for you.

Relationship with Endometriosis

1.
2.
3.
4.
5.
6.

When you begin to think about making a change to the way you approach these situations, you might feel anxious, worried, afraid, or even terrified. Remember, we can bring our compassionate mind to preparing to make a change, as well as making it (see exercise below).

One of the biggest decisions I made in relation to my endometriosis was the decision to have a hysterectomy and excision surgery. Although I knew this would stop my periods and have an impact on my adenomyosis symptoms, I also knew that a hysterectomy was not a cure for endometriosis, so I had no idea what impact it would have on my symptoms associated with that condition. I had chosen a compassionate consultant who was specialised in endometriosis and would perform excision of any endometriosis found. I trusted this consultant completely with my care and was able to connect with compassion from him at this stage in my journey. However, there were no certainties with the surgery, and I read many stories online of other women whose operation did not result in the outcome they had hoped for. I didn't know if it would stop my pain or if it would cause more complications. I used my compassionate mind skills to help me approach the activation of my three systems in relation to my surgery with the qualities of compassion. I imagined myself having the surgery and accepted the support from my compassionate self who reminded me that this surgery was intended to make things better for me. I was able to accept that even if not all my symptoms went away, my periods would stop and the pain from the adenomyosis would stop. You can complete the worksheet below to begin to use your compassionate mind skills to support you to think about making a change that might be helpful to you.

Difficulty (what is the change you are trying to make and how difficult is this for you?)	Before (what steps can you take to prepare for this change? Are there things you could practice to help you tackle this difficulty?)	During (what would be helpful for you to actually make this change or do the thing that is difficult?)	After (what would be helpful for you after you have faced the difficult situation? How might you hold on to any positives? What might help you to tolerate any difficult feelings if it hasn't gone so well? What can you learn from this and do to prevent a setback at this point?)

Now that you have identified the changes you want to make, and a way to approach the initial change, we are going to use imagery to think about making this change. You can use this exercise (adapted from Irons and Beaumont, 2010) for any or all of the changes you want to approach on your list. Start this exercise by connecting with your breathing in a position that is comfortable for you.

> *Bring to mind your compassionate self and its qualities of care, kindness, and commitment to support you. Notice how you feel in this moment when you embody your compassionate self.*
>
> *Now imagine doing one of the changes on your list. Try starting with a situation that is the least anxiety-provoking. Imagine that you are doing this behaviour using the part of you that is strong, wise, and motivated to help you and make things better for you. Notice if any threat or self-criticism shows up when you imagine yourself making this change. If it does, bring your attention back to your compassionate self that is strong and can support you through this fear. Finish by focussing on your soothing rhythm breathing before you open your eyes and connect with the world around you.*

This exercise is aimed to help you guide yourself through making changes in your life. Some of the most significant changes may also be related to decisions about treatment as you manage the impact of endometriosis. In the final part of this chapter, we will think about how to use compassion to aid decision making.

Using Compassion to Make Decisions about Treatment

In chapters 1 and 2, I summarised the many treatments I have received for my problem periods, long before I received a diagnosis of endometriosis. The psychological impact of these treatments has varied from manageable to debilitating. For example, taking the combined pill (the first treatment I received) had a minimal impact on me and helped manage my symptoms; however, GnRH inhibitors (a hormone blocker injection) had a significant impact on my mood, which I could not manage without hormone replacement therapy (HRT). My experience of surgery has been challenging, and some of my hospital admissions have been traumatic. In some ways, my hysterectomy and extensive excision surgery felt like the end of my endometriosis journey, as my life has completely changed since then. However, I still have an ovary and endometriosis symptoms around ovulation, so I know my endometriosis could come back and I may require more treatment in the future. I also continue to come to terms with the impact that endometriosis has had on my life, my identity, and my relationship with the world and other people.

Living with endometriosis brings with it a permanent state of uncertainty. Even when your treatment is controlling your symptoms, you can get caught up in tricky loops wondering what if it stops working or what will happen next. There are many treatment options available, and these are increasing all the time. However, every time you decide about a treatment, you do not know the outcome. Some treatments require you to commit for months at a time, and if they are ineffective, these months can be very difficult – something I experienced with the contraceptive injection and the Mirena coil as these treatments were not effective for me personally. Many people with endometriosis will have multiple surgeries during their journey, which can be both exploratory and/or for treatment purposes. Hospital admissions are common and can be associated with further experiences of not being believed or taken seriously – I had many experiences in hospital of my pain being questioned and often left feeling like I had wasted their time by coming in. I also had experiences where staff were understanding of the severity of my symptoms, and these were helpful and healing for me.

In chapter 2, we discussed the treatments currently available for endometriosis. Any treatment you choose should be discussed with a medical practitioner who can advise you about the advantages of the treatment and any possible side effects or complications that could occur. When you are considering treatments for your endometriosis, it is important to ensure you are fully informed about the treatment and you understand the experience and qualifications of the medical practitioner who will be overseeing this for you. If you have questions or concerns, do not be afraid to ask these, and if you are unhappy or need further assurances, you can ask for a second opinion.

Making difficult decisions about treatment, or questioning the experts, is a place you may find your self-critic show up. Mine would say 'they are the expert, you don't know more than them' or 'you are being a nuisance patient, calling them all the time and going on about your problems when there clearly isn't anything wrong with you'. This would prevent me from advocating for myself, and I sometimes found I was going along with a suggestion that I didn't feel was right for me, just because I didn't feel able to assert myself. As we approach the end of this book, I want to recognise that we are all currently living with a condition that is incurable and we will, therefore, have to continue to make decisions about our treatment and our health throughout our lives. The NHS now recognises the importance of person-centred care which involves keeping the patients views and experience at the centre of the decision making. I hope that this will begin to give us more control and involvement in a process which can often activate our threat systems.

At times when you need to make decisions about your treatment, I would encourage you to look back over chapters 4 and 7. This will bring together the qualities of compassion for you to apply to the decision you have to make. Approach this decision with wisdom, strength, and kindness – I found this then helped me to cope with the treatment afterwards and maintain compassion towards myself if it had not been effective. Remember, compassion means turning towards your suffering and using wisdom to know what to do about it. Being compassionate is itself strong and kind.

To utilise my skills from compassion-focussed work, I found I needed both the wisdom gained from understanding the options available to me and the strength and kindness from myself to make these choices. For me, this meant bringing together facts and information about the treatment options available and then using my compassionate mind to help me navigate those options.

I have put together a two-part guide you can use to navigate treatment decisions. Part 1 covers what you might want to think about prior to a medical appointment and how you can gather information you might need. Part 2 covers how you might use your compassionate mind to navigate the decision you have to make. As you will be familiar with now, I would take a few moments to connect with your soothing rhythm breathing and the qualities of compassion before beginning this exercise.

Part One

What do I need to tell this person today?	What information do I need from this person?	How do I feel about this conversation today?	What might support me to manage my threat system to gain the information I need today?	What can I do after the appointment to help me rebalance?	
I need to tell them that my bleeding and pain are worse than our last appointment.	*I need to know whether any other treatments are available to me now.* *If so, what are they? How might they help me and are there any side effects? Where can I get more information about these treatments to help me make a choice?*	*I can feel my threat system is active as I am worried I will not be listened to or given other treatment options. I am scared it will be another new doctor who will not know my history.*	*I can take my timeline and cycle tracking from chapter 2 to show them if needed.* *I am going to take someone who cares about me to support me.* *I am going to use my soothing rhythm breathing on the drive there and in the waiting room to help me prepare for the appointment.*	*I am going to sit in the car for a few moments and focus on my breath before driving home.* *I am going to write down my first thoughts and feelings so I can reflect on them later.*	

Part Two				
What information did I gain today?	How do I feel in my body when I think about these options? How can I understand this?	What would my compassionate self/other say about the options? How can I approach this decision with wisdom and strength?	What might help me to move forward now?	Are there any skills I can use to help me?
I learnt that I can try hormonal contraceptives to manage my bleeding. I can try a TENS machine to manage my pain in addition to my current pain relief.	*I notice myself feeling tense and anxious. I know this is my threat system being activated because I am worried about trying something new.*	*It is understandable that I am concerned and scared about trying something new that I haven't tried before. I can try this treatment and then make changes if it doesn't work for me — If the treatment does work, I hope it will improve my symptoms.*	*I am going to pick up my prescription and try this. I am going to book a review with the doctor in 8 weeks' time so I know I can speak to them about how the treatment is working for me. I am going to seek out more information about TENS machines using the resources given to me and support networks online.*	*I am going to talk to someone close to me about this decision and ask for their support (chapter 8). I am going to use my skills to support me with my pain. (chapter 9). I am going to think about approaching this change using my compassionate self (chapter 7).*

The aim of this exercise is to bring together the skills from this book to think about treatment decisions during your journey. In my experience, some treatment decisions activate threat more than others. For example, I found the decision to try hormonal contraceptives less threatening, as I knew I could stop taking them if I suffered side effects or found them ineffective. However, treatments that meant committing for a few months activated more threat, as I knew I would be committed to them for a longer period of time. Personally, irreversible decisions such as surgery activated the most threat.

Summary

- Endometriosis has many symptoms, and we may have different relationships with all of them, depending on the impact they have on our lives and the distress we associate with them.
- Endometriosis and fertility can be an area that causes difficult feelings and distress. Although many people with endometriosis do not have difficulties with their fertility, many will experience an activation of threat because fertility difficulties are a possibility. We can use our compassion skills to manage some of the difficult feelings connected with endometriosis and fertility.
- One of the most common symptoms in endometriosis is persistent pain, sometimes called chronic pain. This can be understood by understanding how persistent pain impacts on our three systems. We can then use our compassionate mind skills to connect with compassion in relation to our pain.
- Compassionate behaviour can be a helpful way to connect with compassion. Compassionate behaviour sometimes mean doing something that is challenging for us, and it can be difficult to make these changes. We can use our compassionate mind skills and qualities of compassion to help us plan and make that change.

10 A Commitment to Compassion

Throughout this book, we have focussed on utilising skills from compassion-focussed therapy (CFT) to connect with compassion and reduce the distress you might experience due to living with endometriosis, or the symptoms associated with it. When I set out to write this book, I thought about the impact of the condition and its symptoms across my own journey. I considered both the skills I did use and find helpful, and the skills I feel might have helped me at that time had I been aware of them. I wanted this book to be for anyone who was experiencing difficulties and distress associated with endometriosis, whether your diagnosis is confirmed or not. It takes an average of eight years to receive a confirmed diagnosis in the UK, and I know you could be anywhere along your journey. Wherever you are when you come to the end of this book, I hope it has been helpful for you and that you may revisit it in future at times of challenge for guidance and support.

Perhaps unlike other resources, this book has not focussed on the symptoms of endometriosis or the medical interventions available. As awareness of the condition increases, so do the options for support and treatment which I hope will mean the journey to diagnosis and the experience of living with the disease will improve for people with endometriosis in future. I also hope that compassion and understanding from others increase as we continue to work on reducing the shame and stigma associated with periods, endometriosis, and other gynaecological conditions. However, I believe that whatever treatments become available, some of the emotional distress connected to living with endometriosis is unlikely to go away as it is a difficult condition to manage. This is why I chose to focus this book on the psychological and emotional impact of endometriosis as this was the information I could not access when I was distressed and struggling. Research shows that, like me, 90% of women with endometriosis would have liked access to psychological support but were not offered any (APPG, 2020) I think being unable to access psychological support as part of my NHS healthcare had a negative impact on my experience, and I am grateful that I was able to access this through other avenues including my work and my education. If you can access this as part of your treatment either privately, via the NHS, or through another avenue, I hope this book is a helpful addition to your therapy. If you are not able to access this, I hope this book goes someway to helping you to connect with compassion. Wherever you are in your psychological treatment journey, I want to remind you that I did not always have the knowledge or skills that I have covered in this book, and I continue to work at using my compassionate mind every day. I continually think about and learn to adapt my skills and knowledge to new challenges and difficult feelings. These may be things that you also need to keep working on, and I would encourage you to continue to access support to do this.

In this chapter, I am going to share more of my own journey at the point of ending this book and invite you to bring together your own learning so you can continue to connect with compassion. I will also cover how to access further support in the UK. If you are outside of the UK, you may still find some of the online resources helpful, but there may be other support services in your local area which you may wish to find out more about.

Connecting with Compassion – An Ongoing Commitment

I hope that you have found the resources in this book helpful and have continued to practice them as you have worked through the chapters. I know that when I began exploring different ways of bringing compassion to myself, I could quickly identify how this could help me. However, it took a long time before I started using the skills more regularly, and before they became a part of my life. Like many people,

I looked to learn new skills and ways of coping at times of distress which can make using the skills more difficult. This was one of the biggest challenges in learning new ways of coping in the context of a chronic condition – there might not be a 'good day' to try something new. This doesn't mean that you can't make changes but it may mean that it takes a little longer or is a little more challenging.

I like the analogy of putting up a tent in a storm to think about learning new psychological skills. Let's imagine that you purchase a brand-new tent – it's a large tent, with poles and ropes, and you intend to take it on holiday. You could leave the tent in its bag, drive to your destination, and put the tent up. Now imagine that the tent is quite complicated and difficult because you have never done it before. If it is a nice, sunny day, you have arrived at your destination in plenty of time, you have had a nice journey, stopping for food on the way, then the chances are even if you get a bit stressed, or frustrated, you'll put the tent up. Now imagine it's a windy, wet day – you have had an awful journey that took three times as long as expected, you're hungry, it's late, and getting dark, and you need to put up this complicated tent with all these things working against you. Suddenly, it becomes much less likely that you are going to be able to put that tent up under these difficult conditions and if you do, more likely that you will become very frustrated in the process. However, if you bought the tent and practiced putting it up in your garden a few times before the holiday, then you stand a better chance of being able to erect it whether the weather is sunny or stormy or the journey is good or bad.

Learning psychological skills is a bit like that – you need to practice them as often as you can so you can use them at times of challenge. Ideally, we want to do this on sunny days, but this might not be possible with endometriosis – you may find you are learning to do this in the face of a frequent storm. This doesn't mean you cannot learn how to do this and create some space for yourself – it may mean it takes longer and feels more difficult, but you will be able to get there. Perhaps the task is to find a stormy day which is less like a hurricane or torrential rain, as even though it is not the sunny day we might hope for it may still be possible to practice. The issue with the really stormy days is that your threat system is likely to be so busy that it is harder to think and move towards your wanted outcome of connecting with compassion. The main thing to know is if we want to remember how to put that tent up and keep going on holiday in it, we need to keep practicing how to put it up. Often, we don't do this until we see a reason to, but the more often we practice our skills, the better we will be at using them.

We also know that a tent, although a good form of shelter, may not protect us in the most extreme weather, but it is still likely to be better than no tent at all. As we know, learning the skills we have covered in this book will not stop us from having endometriosis, that is a storm we may continue to weather throughout our lives. However, we may be able to provide ourselves with some shelter from the storm.

My Own Commitment to Connecting with Compassion

My journey with endometriosis has not been one where connecting with compassion has been easy. When I think about the flows of compassion, many of these were missing from my experience. I was fortunate to have compassion from my family and friends, but even those closest to me were not fully aware of my experience because I did not share it with them at that time. I have always tried to offer compassion to others, but I think I sometimes focussed on supporting other people to the detriment of myself. The self-to-self flow of compassion has been an experience of learning a skill in the rain, and this flow is still what I have to work hard on, particularly on stormy days.

Since my hysterectomy and excision surgery, my life has changed completely. I no longer experience many of the symptoms that I have discussed in this book. Although hysterectomy is not a cure for endometriosis, it is a cure for adenomyosis the other condition I was diagnosed with. Hysterectomy also stops your periods, which for me has been a huge relief, and the excision surgery removed the endometriosis that was found throughout my pelvis. However, despite the positive changes that my surgery has had on my life, it is not possible to be cured of endometriosis. I kept an ovary which prevented me from experiencing menopause, and I still have an ovulation cycle because of this. I still have symptoms at these times of the month, particularly migraine, leg pain, and fatigue. I track my cycle so I can be aware of what triggers these symptoms, as whenever I do have pain, I associate this with endometriosis and my threat system is activated. I notice a rush of adrenaline as I try to work out why this symptom is showing up today, and I fear that the severity of symptoms I had before my surgery will be coming back. I live in fear of reaching that level of suffering again. At these times, I connect with my soothing rhythm breathing and bring my compassionate mind online. I remember that these symptoms have an explanation, that I can cope, and if I need help I can access this now. I engage with compassionate behaviour that I would have resisted previously, and I allow the feelings to pass. I find this helps to navigate the physical threat and trauma that I believe will always be present in my body.

I now feel more able to navigate the physical symptoms of threat I experience; however, I still struggle at times with the psychological and the emotional impact living with endometriosis has had on me. I still experience distress connected to the loss and grief that my endometriosis brought into my life. I feel sad that I had to have radical surgery and lose my fertility. I am sad that I endured many traumatic and difficult experiences of healthcare which have impacted my mental health and the way I see the world. I feel angry that I had been told for a long time my symptoms were not worthy of investigation and yet, when I saw the pictures from my surgery and discussed this with my consultant, my endometriosis was widespread and still progressing. I still get caught up in tricky loops that my physical and emotional experiences are not valid. I fear what other people will think about my experiences and my emotions and I still find it hard to open up to others. Writing this book has been a part of my own journey – to openly discuss my experiences not knowing how they will be received.

There are many 'what ifs' in my mind about my past and my future. I often notice my mind wandering to the what ifs in my past and wondering how my life might have been different if I had been diagnosed sooner or received different treatments at different times. My thoughts wander into the future, what if it comes back and less can be done because I have already had radical surgery? What if my daughter suffers like I did? When these times come, I try to bring my focus to the present and ground myself in the now. Connecting with the challenges of my past allows me to connect with compassion and be more open and connected with myself in the present.

As I have talked about in the book, my self-critic has been dominant at many points in my journey. I have believed I am weak, pathetic, and undeserving of compassion. This was, and still is, incredibly painful. When my self-critic is active, or I remember how it was in the past, I remind myself of its function. This helps me to be more compassionate to this part, as I can now connect with a different part, that is a strong, resilient person. I believe I deserve better than the experience I had, and I connect with my compassionate motivation that I want others to have a better experience than I did. I believe that increasing awareness of the value of compassion and of CFT will improve the experience of living with endometriosis for many people in future. I am able to connect with the flow of self-to-self compassion and know it is OK that I still feel many difficult emotions because of endometriosis. I am also more able to connect with compassion from others which has had a positive impact on the relationships that I value in my life. I have been able to let go of relationships that have been unhelpful to me in the past.

I feel that I am more able to seek out support and compassion from others and not to run away if I do not receive a compassionate response, but instead be able to remember that this experience is not representative of all my experiences. Being able to share my journey is part of connecting with compassion from others – naming and taming the shame I have carried in the hope it will not continue to survive both for me personally but also for other women and menstruating people in the future. I find value in being able to give compassion to others, and I hope this book has brought some compassion to you. This book has allowed me to experience all three flows of compassion as I have revisited many painful parts of my journey – it has been a process for me, one that is ongoing. I have benefitted from writing it more than I imagined, but my motivation was and remains to provide compassion for you and give you the skills to connect with compassion yourself. I hope you can continue this journey with compassion, wherever your endometriosis journey takes you.

Your Commitment to Connecting with Compassion

As you develop your skills and your awareness of yourself and your own needs, I hope it will become easier to use them at times of high distress. When I experienced some of my most severe flare-ups, it would have been impossible to use some of the skills in this book; however, I always found it helpful to use my soothing rhythm breathing and coping statements that came from my compassionate self. This took a lot of energy to use these skills, and I had to focus my mind on them as it would often be distracted by intense pain – but going back to the present, my breath and my coping statements helped me to survive those moments of acute distress and retain a sense of control.

There may be times when you experience other setbacks in trying to connect with compassion. These might be unrelated to your endometriosis but might still make it hard to utilise the skills we have learnt in this book, such as stress at work, financial stressors, relationship difficulties, or bereavement. It might also be things related to your endometriosis, such as surgeries or flare-ups. It can be helpful to spend some time thinking about the possible challenges and setbacks you might face in the future and how you might cope with these. This is part of the commitment we make to staying compassionate, wise, and strong in the face of the challenges we may encounter in the future.

Let's take some time to reflect on what you have learnt in this book, the changes you have made, the things you want to continue to work on, and how you might continue to connect with your compassionate self at times of challenge. Like all the exercises in this book, it may first be helpful to connect with your soothing rhythm breathing and the qualities of your compassionate self as being committed to caring for you, with wisdom and strength. I am not going to guide you through this preparation, as I hope you are now able to connect with this yourself before completing the worksheet below.

Endometriosis and Me
What have I learnt about how endometriosis impacts me and my life?
What have I learnt about how I see myself? How does this show up for me?
What have I been able to change since reading this book?
What do I still find difficult?
When I find things hard, what can I do to connect with the three flows of compassion?

Once you have completed this plan, I suggest that you take a picture so you can keep these ideas with you and refer to them. It is likely that you will continue to update and change this in response to different events and circumstances. Some people I have worked with in therapy print out these plans and put them on their fridge or by a desk so they will see them frequently and be reminded of their commitment to themselves. Other people keep them on their phone or make them into a small card they can carry around with them. As always, do whatever works for you.

How to Get More Support

As we have covered, this book is intended to help you along your journey with endometriosis and connect with compassion. However, there are many other resources and organisations also available to help and support you. I am going to close this book with a list of helpful organisations that are available. You will also find a reference list at the end of the book if you wish to explore any of the resources further. The resources and support available for endometriosis and for CFT continue to grow. I hope that through this book, and the investment and development of endometriosis treatment and communities, you can find the resources you need to connect with compassion and reduce your distress.

I hope that you can utilise everything we have learnt together and the support that is available to continue your journey with strength, wisdom, and kindness. Thank you.

Resources

Mental Health Concerns

Endometriosis can have an impact on mental health. There is an identified link between endometriosis and mental health conditions such as depression and anxiety (Koller et al, 2023). Living with endometriosis can lead to new mental health difficulties that you didn't have before or impact mental health difficulties that were already part of your experience. Throughout this book we have thought about lots of these feelings and behaviours. We might all have experienced them at some point in our journey. However, if you are experiencing these symptoms most or all of the time, feeling stuck in these symptoms or unable to move forward then you might benefit from some more support with your mental health.

Symptoms of Depression
- Feeling down or hopeless
- Little interest or pleasure in things you usually enjoy
- Feeling bad about yourself
- Feeling irritable
- Feeling tired, lacking energy
- Difficulty concentrating
- Difficulty sleeping or wanting to sleep all the time
- Loss of appetite or overeating
- Thoughts of suicide or of not wanting to be around

Symptoms of Anxiety
- Feeling nervous or anxious
- Difficulty relaxing
- Ongoing worrying thoughts
- Worrying about lots of different things
- Fearing the worst
- Feeling irritable
- Feeling restless or agitated

If these symptoms sound like something you are experiencing, then I would recommend you seek further support. We have talked in this book about how difficult it can be to seek support from healthcare professionals as a person with endometriosis, as you may have had repeated experiences of not feeling listened to. However, your mental health, like your physical health, is important, and if you need support and treatment it is important that you ask for it. Hopefully you know now from this book and any other support you are receiving that you are not alone, you can talk to people about the help you need and that there is help available for you.

Where to Seek Further Support

1. You may be able to access psychological therapy or counselling via your GP or local well-being service. Sometimes these services are called IAPT teams (Improving access to psychological therapies) or NHS talking therapies or well-being services. Sometimes they are called something else. You can self-refer to these services if you know what they are called in your local area. These services offer short-term counselling and therapies to people experiencing common mental health difficulties. In the UK, these services are expanding to also cover some long term health conditions. More information can be found on the NHS website. However, it you don't know what services are available in your area or don't think this will be the right service for you, it is likely to be helpful to start with your GP as they will have the best knowledge of what mental health support is available.
2. If you are under the care of a specialist endometriosis service, they may have access to a clinical, counselling or health psychologist. These are highly trained and regulated practitioner psychologists who are trained to work with people struggling with the emotional impact of physical health problems. If you are experiencing significant emotional difficulties, then you may be referred to a qualified psychologist within the specialist team.
3. If you wish to see a psychologist privately, it is important to ensure you see someone who is highly trained and regulated. The term 'psychologist' is not a protected title. Therefore, you should seek someone who is registered with the Health & Care Professions Council (HCPC). Anyone calling themselves a clinical, health or counselling psychologist should be registered with HCPC. You can check the register on the HCPC website.

For more on finding a clinical psychologist, the Association of Clinical Psychologists UK (ACP-UK) has a useful guide on its website.

If you are at risk to yourself

As stated above, thoughts of suicide or not wanting to be around can be an indication of depression. If you notice any of the below symptoms, then you should seek immediate help:–

Being preoccupied with thoughts of death or dying
Making a plan of how you would end your life
Taking steps to say goodbye to loved ones
Acquiring things to follow through your plan
Writing a suicide note

Where to Seek Further Crisis Support
1. It is important to let your GP know about any of these symptoms. Ask for an urgent appointment.
2. If you live in England, you can access the NHS Urgent Mental Health helpline via the NHS website. There is also a mental health text support service which you can access by texting SHOUT to 85258.
3. The Samaritans are trained to support people who are feeling suicidal. You can call them for free at any time on 116 123. There are also other ways to get in touch with the Samaritans on their website.
4. If you are concerned that you are at high or immediate risk of suicide then you should go to the Accident & Emergency Department at your local hospital. There will be a psychiatric liaison team on duty who will be able to assess you and work with you to develop an immediate plan to support you.

Resources for Endometriosis and Other Gynaecological Conditions

There are a wide range of resources on many of the topics in this book available from Endometriosis UK www.endometriosis-uk.org – support includes online information, helplines, local support groups, web chat, and an online community.
The NHS website provides information about the condition: www.nhs.uk/conditions/endometriosis. Information about adenomyosis can also be accessed via this website.
The Menstrual Health Project provides a wide range of information sheets about a range of gynaecological conditions including endometriosis. They also provide webinars and education to increase awareness and reduce stigma.
The Royal College of Obstetricians and Gynaecologists (RCOG) has several information sheets for women/people who menstruate and information for professionals.

CFT Resources

You can access a wide range of resources from The Compassionate Mind Foundation https://www.compassionatemind.co.uk/
Several exercises in this book are adapted from The Compassionate Mind Workbook (Irons and Beaumont, 2017) https://www.compassionatemind.co.uk/resource/books

Relationship Support and Resources

Women's Aid provide information and support on domestic abuse information and support on domestic abuse (womensaid.org.uk)
Refuge offer a National Domestic Abuse Helpline in the UK and further information via their website (nationaldahelpline.org.uk)
Relate offer couples therapy and relationship support in the UK. Information about what is available in your local area can be found on their website.

Employment Support and Resources

Endometriosis UK have guidance for dealing with endometriosis at work which can be accessed via the website. The document is called: Hints and tips for dealing with employers (New Branding).pdf (endometriosis-uk.org)

In the UK, the Department for Work and Pensions offer support and advice about employment via their website - GOV.UK (www.gov.uk)

Fertility Support and Resources

Both of the following websites offer support and advice around fertility:

Fertility Network UK: https://fertilitynetworkuk.org/
Fertility Friends - www.fertilityfriends.co.uk

Baby Loss Charities

Some people will experience pregnancy or baby loss during their journey. The following organisations and websites offer further support for loss in the UK.

Tommys: https://www.tommys.org/
Petals: https://petalscharity.org/
Miscarriage Association: https://www.miscarriageassociation.org.uk/

References

Adamson, G. D., Kennedy, S. H., and Hummelshoj, L. (2010). Creating solutions in endometriosis: Global collaboration through the World Endometriosis Research Foundation. *Journal of Endometriosis* 2:3–6.

All Party Parliamentary Group (2020). Endometriosis in the UK: Time for change. *APPG on Endometriosis Inquiry Report*. All-Party Parliamentary Group on Endometriosis — Nuffield Department of Women's & Reproductive Health (ox.ac.uk).

Always (retrieved 2023). *Period Stigma around the world today*. Period Stigma Around the World | Always®.

Ballard, K. D., Lowton, K., and Wright, J. T. (2006). What's the delay? A qualitative study of women's experiences of reaching a diagnosis of endometriosis. *Fertility and Sterility* 86:1296–1301.

BBC News (2019). *Sex education: Menstrual health to be taught in schools by 2020*. Sex education: Menstrual health to be taught in school by 2020 – BBC News.

BBC News (2021). *Women in 20s told to 'get pregnant' to ease endometriosis symptoms*. Women in 20s told 'get pregnant' to ease endometriosis symptoms – BBC News.

Borrell-Carrió, F., Suchman, A. L., and Epstein, R. M. (2004). The biopsychosocial model 25 years later: Principles, practice, and scientific inquiry. *Annals of Family Medicine* 2(6):576–582. doi: 10.1370/afm.245. PMID: 15576544; PMCID: PMC1466742.

Brene Brown, RSA Short (2013) *Brene Brown on Empathy*.https://www.youtube.com/watch?v=1Evwgu369Jw

Brene Brown (2013) https://brenebrown.com/articles/2013/01/15/shame-v-guilt/

Brown, B. (2015). *Daring greatly: How the courage to be vulnerable transforms the way we live, love, parent, and lead*. Avery.

Brown, K. S. (2007). Dyspareunia due to endometriosis: A qualitative study of its effect on the couple relationship (Dissertation). *ProQuest Information & Learning*.

References

BUPA (retrieved 2023). *Endometriosis as work*. Endometriosis at work | Women's Health Hub | Bupa UK.

Butt, F., and Chesla, C. (2007). Relational patterns of couples living with chronic pelvic pain from endometriosis. *Qualitative Health Research* 17:571–585.

Dale-Hewitt, V., & Irons, C. (2015). Compassion Focused Therapy. In D. L. Dawson, N. G. Moghaddam (Eds) *Formulation in Action*, 161.

Department for Work and Pensions (2023). Department for Work and Pensions – GOV.UK (www.gov.uk).

Department of Health (2022). *Results of the "Women's Health – Let's talk about it survey"*. Results of the 'Women's Health – Let's talk about it' survey – GOV.UK (www.gov.uk).

Doyle, M., and Carballedo, A. (2014). Infertility and mental health. *Advances in Psychiatric Treatment* 20(5):297–303. doi: 10.1192/apt.bp.112.010926.

Endometriosis Awareness Month 2020 launches to tackle the fact 54% don't know about endometriosis | Endometriosis UK (endometriosis-uk.org).

Endometriosis UK – Menstrual wellbeing to be taught in schools by 2020 | Endometriosis UK (endometriosis-uk.org).

Endometriosis UK, 2022 – Endometriosis facts and figures | Endometriosis UK (endometriosis-uk.org).

Endometriosis UK (2022). What is endometriosis? | Endometriosis UK (endometriosis-uk.org).

Endometriosis UK, 2023a– Endometriosis UK - Endometriosis, Fertility and Pregnancy Jan 2023.pdf (endometriosis-uk.org)

Endometriosis UK, 2023 – Endometriosis UK – Endometriosis, fertility and pregnancy Jan 2023.pdf (endometriosis-uk.org).

Engel, G. L. (1977). The need for a new medical model: A challenge for biomedicine. *Science* 196(4286):129–136. doi: 10.1126/science.847460. PMID: 847460.

Equality Act 2010 (Commencement No.3) Order 2010, S.I. 2010/2317 § 2 (2010). https://www.legislation.gov.uk/uksi/2010/2317/madeParenthetical Citation.

Facchin, F., Barbara, G., Dridi, D., Alberico, D., Buggio, L., Somigliana, E., Saita, E., and Vercellini, P. (2017). Mental health in women with endometriosis: Searching for predictors of psychological distress. *Human Reproduction* 32(9). doi: 10.1093/humrep/dex249.

Gilbert, P. (1998). What is shame? Some core issues and controversies. In P. Gilbert and B. Andrews (Eds.), *Shame: Interpersonal behavior, psychopathology and culture* (pp. 3–38). Oxford University Press. (SHAME DEFINITION).

Gilbert -.P ., (2014) https://self-compassion.org/wp-content/uploads/publications/GilbertCFT.pdf

Gilbert, P., & Miles, J. (Eds.) (2002). *Body shame: Conceptualisation, research & treatment*. Routledge

References

Gilbert, P. (2010a). *The compassionate mind.* Constanble. ISBN-10: 1849010986.

Gilbert, P. (2014). The origins and nature of compassion focussed therapy. *British Journal of Clinical Psychology*, 53: 6–41.

Gilbert, P., and Miles, J. (Eds.). (2002). *Body shame: Conceptualisation, research & treatment.* Routledge.

Hennegan, J., Winkler, I. T., Bobel, C., Keiser, D., Hampton, J., Larsson, G., Chandra-Mouli, V., Plesons, M., and Mahon, T. (2021). Menstrual health: A definition for policy, practice and research. *Sexual and Reproductive Health Matters* 29(1). doi: 10.1080/26410397.2021.1911618.

Hill, M. (2019). *Period power.* Bloomsbury Publishing.

Hudson, N., Culley, L., Law, C., Mitchell, H., Denny, E., and Raine-Fenning, N. (2016). 'We needed to change the mission statement of the marriage': Biographical disruptions, appraisals and revisions among couples living with endometriosis. *Sociology of Health and Illness* 38:721–735.

Irons, C., and Beaumont, E. (2017). *The compassionate mind workbook. A step-by-step guide to compassion focussed therapy.* Robinson Publishing.

Johnson, N. P., Hummelshoj, L., Adamson, G. D., Keckstein, J., Taylor, H. S., Abrao, M. S., Bush, D., Kiesel, L., Tamimi, R., Sharpe-Timms, K. L., Rombauts, L., and Giudice, L. C. (2017). World Endometriosis Society Sao Paulo Consortium. World Endometriosis Society consensus on the classification of endometriosis. *Human Reproduction* 32(2):315–324. doi: 10.1093/humrep/dew293.

Kunz, G., Beil, D., Huppert, P., Noe, M., Kissler, S., and Leyendecker, G. (2005). Adenomyosis in endometriosis–prevalence and impact on fertility. Evidence from magnetic resonance imaging. *Human Reproduction* 20(8):2309–2316. doi: 10.1093/humrep/dei021.

Lee, S. Y., Koo, Y. J., and Lee, D. H. (2021). Classification of endometriosis. *Yeungnam University Journal of Medicine* 38(1):10–18. doi: 10.12701/yujm.2020.00444.

Leyendecker, G., Bilgicyildirim, A., Inacker, M., Stalf, T., Huppert, P., Mall, G., Bottcher, B., and Wildt, L. (2015). Adenomyosis and endometriosis. Re-visiting their association and further insights into the mechanisms of auto-traumatisation. An MRI study. *Archives of Gynecology and Obstetrics* 291(4). doi: 10.1007/s00404-014-3437-8.

Linton, S. J., and Shaw, W. S. (2011). Impact of psychological factors in the experience of pain. *Physical Therapy* 91(5):700–711. doi: 10.2522/ptj.20100330.

Maddern, J., Grundy, L., Castro, J., and Brierley, S. M. (2020). Pain in endometriosis. *Frontiers in Cellular Neuroscience* 14:590823. doi: 10.3389/fncel.2020.590823.

Meuleman, C., Vandenabeele, B., Fieuws, S., Spiessens, C., Timmerman, D., and D'Hooghe, T. (2009). High prevalence of endometriosis in infertile women with normal ovulation and normospermic partners. *Fertility and Sterility* 92(1):68–74. doi: 10.1016/j.fertnstert.2008.04.056.

Michas, F. (2022). Registered doctors by gender and specialty in the UK 2021 | Statista.

NHS UK. (2023a). Adenomyosis – NHS (www.nhs.uk).

NHS Website (2023b) https://www.nhs.uk/mental-health/conditions/depression-in-adults/symptoms/

NHS Website (2023c) https://www.nhs.uk/every-mind-matters/mental-health-issues/anxiety/#signs-of-anxiety

NHS. (2022a). Periods – NHS (www.nhs.uk).

NHS. (2022b). Endometriosis – NHS (www.nhs.uk).

NICE Guideline [NG73]: Endometriosis Diagnosis and Management (2017). https://www.nice.org.uk/guidance/ng73.

Penlington, C. (2018). Exploring a compassion focused intervention for persistent pain in a group setting. *British Journal of Pain* 13(1). doi: 10.1177/2049463718772148.

Plan International UK (2018). Break the barriers: Girls experience of menstruation in the UK. download (plan-uk.org).

Rios, G. R. *The importance of menstrual health education.* The Importance of Menstrual Health Education – Girls' Globe (girlsglobe.org).

Roth, T. (1998). Getting on clinical training courses. *The Psychologist, December*, pp. 589–592.

Royal College of Nursing (2021). Fertility has a huge emotional impact on people's lives. 'Fertility has a huge emotional impact on people's lives' | RCN Magazines | Royal College of Nursing.

Royal College of Nursing (2022). Promoting menstrual wellbeing. *Clinical Professional Resource.*

Royal College of Psychiatrists Perinatal mental health services: What are they? | Royal College of Psychiatrists (rcpsych.ac.uk).

Schick, M., Germeyer, A., Bottcher, B., Hecht, S., Geiser, M., Rosner, S., Eckstein, M., Vomstein, K., Toth, B., Strowitzki, T., Wischmann, T., and Ditzen, B. (2022). Partners matter: The psychosocial well-being of couples when dealing with endometriosis. *Health and Quality of Life Outcomes* 20:86. doi: 10.1186/s12955-022-01991-1.

Schluter, C., Kragg, G., and Schmidt, J. (2023). Body Shaming: An exploratory study on its definition and classification. *International Journal of Bullying Prevention* 5. doi: 10.1007/s42380-021-00109-3.

Schneiderman, N., Ironson, G., and Siegel, S. D. (2005). Stress and health: Psychological, behavioral, and biological determinants. *Annual Review of Clinical Psychology* 1:607–628. doi: 10.1146/annurev.clinpsy.1.102803.144141. PMID: 17716101; PMCID: PMC2568977.

References

Soo-Young, L., Koo, Y., and Dae-Hyung, L. (2021). Classification of endometriosis. *Yeungnam University Journal of Medicine* 38(1). doi: 10.12701/yujm.2020.00444.

The compassionate mind foundation, 2023 – Compassionate Mind Foundation.

The Pain Toolkit (2023). Definition of persistent pain. https://www.paintoolkit.org/what-is-pain

Young, K., Fisher, J., and Kirkman, M. (2015). Women's experiences of endometriosis: A systematic review and synthesis of qualitative research. *Journal of Family and Reproductive Health Care* 41(3):225–234. doi: 10.1136/jfprhc-2013-100853. Epub 2014 Sep 2. PMID: 25183531.

About the Author

Dr Kirsty Harris is a consultant clinical psychologist working within the NHS in Mental Health Services. Kirsty is passionate about working with women and women's health. Kirsty first learnt about compassion-focussed therapy during her clinical psychology training at Oxford University. She has since integrated this approach into both her professional work and her personal life, as a woman with endometriosis. In this book, Kirsty shares her experiences of living with the symptoms of endometriosis and the impact it has had on her life with the hope that this can make a difference to women and menstruating people like herself.

www.ingramcontent.com/pod-product-compliance
Lightning Source LLC
Chambersburg PA
CBHW051544020426
42333CB00016B/2089